Barkin' Dog

How to Talk with Aphasia

By

Ed Bas

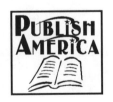

PublishAmerica
Baltimore

First printing

ISBN: 1-4137-3062-0
PUBLISHED BY PUBLISHAMERICA, LLLP
www.publishamerica.com
Baltimore

Printed in the United States of America

For my son, Derek
and
my daughter, Shannon

"It is good to have an end to journey toward,
but it is the journey that matters, in the end."
Ursula LeGuin

A writer has to write a book, at least one life. This one is mine. I had a stroke from resulting aphasia with my years to write about them. I learned at aphasia with few books for me to read. I learned a lot, learning from the Internet, pamphlets and conversations with therapists and patients. But a little from books. I had a bad life after my stroke. I had a good life, just like everybody's life. I had a divorce just into the pre- and post-stroke. I was losing my wife – almost even my children. I lost my job. I even lost my communication. That was really hard because I am a writer and an editor, a communicator for words. There are also degrees of aphasia between mild and severe. A person may speak only in single words or in short, fragmented phrases. I learned to write, and read and speak – a little. It's what a book publisher and a reader really wants! I've taken away my life, from educating to exercising. But I had to learn myself, and questioned to many people. I read a lot of books in writing this book: not just stroke and aphasia, but science and technology, speech and language therapy, exercise, jobs, computers, medicine and government benefits. I learned, just as had to learn for myself – a stumble, a blunder. I tried, and failed. Readers don't have to try and fail. They can succeed, without my mistakes. In this book was a second effort, not only for my readers. As writing my book, it was sort of a speech-language therapy. Looking at it, it was a pre-stroke life and a life of post-stroke. I wrote many of my dead ends. I've had to contact many of my friends, therapists, government officials, employees-employers and insurance agents. Too many doctors, neurologists, cardiologists – and their collection agencies! Aphasia turned my life topsy-turvy. One day is different from one day last year, or it will be five years pre-stroke. All stroke patients can learn – and they can master it from their lives and my life.

Table of Contents

Book One

Book Two

All my family, friends, acquaintances, patients, instructors and doctors are real persons. I didn't write imagined people, and no pseudonyms. As a journalist, I wrote their real names. They are all kind, and were always courageous. Truth is the best thing. If they were still occasionally misquoted without my notes, I apologize. But it's my life, and their words are also mine.

Barkin' Dog
How to Talk with Aphasia

by Ed Bas

"What is the use of a book," thought Alice,
"without pictures or conversations?"
Alice's Adventures in Wonderland

'Twas brillig. and the slithy toves
Did gyre and gimble in the wabes
All mimsy were the borogroves,
And the mome raths outgrabe."
Jabberwocky

Book One

Chapter 1

A difficult career

Stroke was a difficult and utmost failure for my journalism career.

What is the use of a book, or a journalist, without conversations?

I had a stroke in June 2002. That was only a single moment, one that opened my life, the dismal gates of hell for "the use of a book without... conversations." My heart failed once again (and *only* again). My career lasted 26 years, from the college at the time of 1975. It almost ended a life, much of a career. It was a sudden stop as it was for me, like the whooooshing of a train. Editor and publisher, the double whammy, I was trying to understand words at the thesaurus at a computer. I tried a dozen words. The words were correct, but they were elusive from me. There was a long for six months prior to my stroke.

It was a disappointing time to end 19 years of marriage. My six months, or a year or two years, of pain wasn't the stroke – it was my heart throbbing. My wife filed the papers for a divorce. My life was ending at my divorce and my stroke.

What was I doing there? What was I doing here, 13 months after then? I was in a summer camp for a weekend in the Thumb of Michigan with the Stroke Association, an American Heart Association. It was a YWCA Camp Cavell, along the pristine woods for Lake Huron. I was in a crowd of victims, blacks and whites, all adult ages but mostly the age of 60s and 70s. They sleep in log cabins with cots, a lodge and meals prepared from volunteers. I was there among them, there were stroke survivors. I still haven't my voice, or at least sentences, after post-year. I was only saying words, individually and combined, two or three words or short sentences. "Hi! How are you doing?" Some people just smiled, or nodded their heads. We said it every hour, every chance. I was really lucky. I don't worry for an injured arm and a leg, with a walker or cane, or with a distorted vision. At a "beach party" it was a pity. I had a bad feeling for "our" survivors. So many are in their wheelchairs, and walking or stumbling with canes. Jon was my age. He told me about his life, at a pleasant day on the sandy beach at Camp Cavell, on a clear sapphire sky and a temperature in the mid-80s. Jon had a job at Home Depot, the home repair store, but he once was an instructor at a college, flew an airplane as a pilot and had a degree in financing and economics – a busy, enlightening life. He had 12 years ago a heart attack and quickly a stroke. It's a terrible pity, and a terrible lifetime. At least he had a wife, Julia. He was married, I was divorced. Jon is lucky. She is a handy masseuse for the campers. "I am still alive!" he said, once or twice. "I'm grateful for my life." With a happy-go-lucky, he struggled volleyball serving with one good arm, and a really good volleyball game with survivors and YMCA-YWCA therapists and volunteers.

All of them are happy, and living every day and night. They have families, and among them have them for the weekend – kids, grandchildren, brothers and sisters. We had a talent show: danced, sang and talked corny jokes. We dined together, breakfast or lunch or dinner. We ate s'mores at the campfire – marshmallows and graham crackers and candy bars – roasting in the campfires. There was very little fat served in the meals, or reduced cholesterol with lean chicken or hamburgers or veggie-burgers if you wanted them, with salads and fruit with every meal. "Do you want some help? Can you walk with your cane?" We told each other how frustrating it is communicating with aphasia, and how it had a tough time with after having a stroke within a year, or 10 years. On Saturday afternoon we had a beach party, and Saturday evening we played cards or volleyball (no alcohol and almost prohibited smoking tobacco). On Sunday morning we sang songs and prayed aloud for each other. They are the stroke survivors, and the stroke victors. But what was I doing then or there, my very first Camp Cavell? Did I really have a stroke? Was I a survivor? You betcha. Why will I be there after one year, or after five years or ten years? I really don't understand what gave me a life with a stroke. I understand maybe, but I am frustrating and angry. My words and my voice don't communicate, don't vocalize after one year or two years post-stroke. It's hard after you lost your words. Like a dog, but dogs don't care – barkin' dog!

Twelve months ago, I probably drank too much. My wife surprised me, telling me that she wasn't happy during the past 10 years, and it was no reason for counseling. She won't be married to me even for six months. A couple of days of drinking beer and running and biking, after 25 miles on bike, then four miles of running, maybe it made me dehydrated for a hot summer day. I was tired, depressed, thirsty? There were reasons for a stroke. Maybe, maybe, maybe... It was not at a hard task on Saturday when I was working at home. I was routing the cable t.v. for 14-year-old Shannon's bedroom from an additional bedroom as an office-computer room.

My son Derek, 17, was at home that day, and helped my life. He phoned 911. He felt the old Dad was sleeping too much! I took a nap on the bedroom in the middle of rerouting a t.v. cable, but I couldn't get awake. There was no pain at all, not hurting. When the ambulance crew came in (probably 10 minutes), I was conscious, but I was both awake and unconscious. Falling asleep, I noticed the drive taking the ambulance at an unfamiliar hospital. It was a short drive that took another 10 minutes. I was eventually checking out the hospital, 10 days later in for a deep, spooky, eerie, funky life.

I was gone for 10 days in St. John Macomb Hospital in Warren, Michigan, but after I was leaving with 100% physical condition. I had the usual tests. No operations, no stitches, no cuts or scalpels. I felt like I could run a couple of miles. I ran every daily afterwards. It took me two miles, then three or four for every single day. I was biking, walking and tennis with my son Derek, I would exercise daily. I had an exercise regularly which I had time. My mind wasn't practical, so it was time for the body to actively exercise. I couldn't write, read or talk.

Every male with a stroke will have a 47% chance within five years. One in five Americans will have a stroke. From the word, *aphasia*: loss or impairment of the power to use or comprehend words usually resulting from brain damage.

"Although a variety of language disorders had been recognized prior to the mid-nineteenth century, the study of aphasia can be directly can be directly traced to the work of a 37-year-old surgeon and anthropologist Paul Pierre Broca," wrote Carl Sagan in his book, *Broca's Brain*.

Paul Broca was a surgeon, a neurologist and an anthropologist. He was a scientist and developed both medicine and anthropology 150 years. Broca "performed distinguished work on cancer pathology and the treatment of aneurysms, and made a landmark contribution to understanding the origins of aphasia – an impairment of the ability to articulate ideas." The German neurologist Wernicke described symptoms and location in the late 1800s. It is one of the most worst of aphasics, unable to repeat your words.

My mind felt it was helpless. I could think and I couldn't speak. "Imagine being trapped inside your own mind, unable to effectively communicate with the rest of humanity," wrote the *Stroke Smart* trade magazine. "These fears have served as adaptive and useful function in the past. But I believe they are mostly emotional baggage in the present. I was interested, as a scientist who had written about the brain, to find such revulsion hiding in me, to be revealed for my inspection in Broca's collection. These fears are worth fighting for."

I thought, how can I work? If, for example, even I was a heat and cooling service technician, which I mostly write about contractors for trade magazines. A stroke's conditions would not prohibit the rigorous tasks from these jobs. I could drive a service van. I could read my service orders. I could do the work and talk with the customers and friends, then a couple of hours either as at a warehouse or at a headquarters. But my "sense of speaking" had stolen my voice. I was able to communicate a little. As we know, the effects of stroke on each individual person are different. Some people with aphasia continue to improve over time. Others get little return in the way of speaking. But it was tough to talk for 15 minutes, or to ask them an explanation for their work, like a reporter. My real job.

I was 100% disabled.

My speaking isn't terrible – *really*. I could buy gasoline for the van and coffee break (milk, not sugar), then discuss for friendly employees, take directions with a dispatcher, and order for lunch... for three or four words, but not much. I can speak sentences if they're shorter. "I have had a stroke, and it is hard for me to speak, read and write. I usually understand what is said, but it helps if you speak clearly. Your help and patience would be appreciated. Thank you." That's a card in my wallet behind my driver's license. Cops don't read it. I know that. They don't care. But it makes an interesting tip so you don't have to say, "I ...have...no, I had... a...*(ummm)* stroke."

I had a guardian and a conservator, helping a hand and keeping my money and bills. That was my guardian and she is my sister, Ann. Sometimes she wanted to get my financing or my divorce, but she was not exactly what I wished for or wanted to. It was my fault, trying to communicate for my purposes. It was a three-words or four-words sentence that sounds like a vocal telegraph. "I will go... *stop*... to the store... *stop*... with my car..." Aphasia is a common complication of stroke, head injuries, tumors and infections. There are a million people who have aphasia. I am reclaiming my speech from a language disorder that affects a person's ability to produce and comprehend speech, as well as writing and reading. Four components of decision-making capacity:

Understanding – ability to comprehend diagnosis and treatment information; what is wrong, what is wrong, what are the alternative treatments, what are the risks and benefits.

Appreciation – what does all of the information mean for the patient; does the patient believe the diagnosis, and appreciate that recommendations might benefit him/her.

Reasoning – patient is able to think through the choices in a way that is logical or consistent with his/her core values.

Expressing a choice – patient is able to reach a decision and communicate it.

My career was my talking, writing and reading. Aphasia is one subject. I talked to a friend, Doris, who I said, "Doesn't it sound like fantasy? As though it means a fantasy instead of language." Many medical words are suffering: heart attack, stroke, cancer, diverticulitis, anthrax, poxvirus... not like *aphasia!* It's a handicap, with a lost arm or your eyes blinded. Words for a simple sentence, but you try to cut to only two words or three words. *Go car.* What? Say it again? Or *"go to the car."* In other words, "It's time to go to the car for a ride at the supermarket." Look! It's 13 words, a lot of "for, the, in, a, at." It seems simple. But "time, car, persons, ride" means a little sentence without so many prepositions and adjectives and adverbs. Try to make it understood, without so many words. Cut 13 words to two, or three. It's feasible but occasionally it's scrambled or harder to understand. Go car? You mean, "someone stole your car?"

At the same time, aphasia is a word that people cannot pronounce. People who have had strokes have an even harder time pronouncing it: a-fa-zh. All that people who will make it even harder, then make it difficult to people with a stroke. Neurologist Dr. Lionel Glass said to me, "Go it's easy. Take it slow. Take the words slowly for what you want to say." As though it's easy a sentence. You never take the time, you never say, "Oh, I'll just take the time for people to understand me." It's easy from him. The words are not very complicated. They are simple. Taking them enough time and having a thesaurus on your brain does not make it effortlessly. If you have paper and a pen for those who will take those for words. As though it's your mouth and throat won't say your words. You can say it, once you can correct ones in your computer – delete, insert, save as, etc. I can read what's in front of my eyes. "Also, unfortunately, many physicians know very little neurology and even less about brain function," said writers Cleo Hutton and Louis Caplan, "Striking Back at Stroke." That's true. Many neurologists know very little neurology. Doctors can explain the intestines, liver, stomach, kidneys, even the heart and arteries and blood vessels but they don't understand how or why or what explains a brain. How does the brain put together the separate motor systems, vision, hearing, feeling, neurons, speech, and memory? If doctors and researchers can't say it, how can writers write the central nervous system or the brain?

"I keep instructions and explanations simple. Speak slowly but naturally. Do not shout or speak loudly." That was the first of 33 written speech-language family suggestions for pathology communicating with a stroke patient. I told it was too many. That "family" would not listen to 33 suggestions, no matter how they are well intended. It's probably any family who would read the 33 suggestions, more than attempting to understand the stroke patient.

But some are good and true. Second: don't put the patient on display or force them to speak. Third: don't discuss the patient's problem in front of him/her. Always assume they can understand everything. Fourth: help the patient maintain their former status in the family group. Include them in family affairs as much as possible.

#5 – Don't discuss outside problems that may be stressful to patient unless it's absolutely necessary.

#6 – Have a positive attitude. Praise each sign of progress in speech and language as it occurs. Emphasize their abilities, not their disabilities in language.

#7 – Create a relaxed atmosphere by never appearing to be hurried or anxious yourself. Give the patient an attitude of acceptance.

#8 – Allow time for the patient to understand what you are saying and time to react. It takes longer after a stroke.

#9 – Explain what has happened to the patient. Repeat this often because they may not understand the first time or they might forget. Give simple explanations.

#10 – Usually the easiest way for a patient to respond is to "fill in the blank," e.g. It was a cup of _____.

My favorite was #21: If the patient is an adult, *treat them as an adult*. The patient has not lost their intelligence but rather their ability to communicate effectively. I'm afraid to "lost" my intelligence. To ruin your own ability to communicate, also loses some of your intelligence.

Chapter 2

Aphasia meeting

Ya gotta be ready for the fastball.
Ted Williams

At women's conference room within the St. Joseph Hospital in Macomb County, a meeting of 14 persons talked about the subject of aphasia. They talked and gestured. It seemed like a few birds, chirping at the dawn. Like they just learned to talk, and want to make it as long as it will take. But three or four are reluctant, or really don't say much at all. It's communication on a merry-go-round. It continually goes 'round, like a circle. When you want to make it stop, or want at least ticket to your body, you feel it's quicker and a blur. You want to say it aloud, or silent: it's your choice. To communicate or not?

It's better sometimes to keep silent. If you make an effort to make one, it tries to put out three and four words to make a sentence, which requires 10 words to work. I can try for a noun, a verb, maybe an adjective. "Drive to big store." That means I drive with my van to Meijer's grocery, perfect. Then aphasics understand, and nod his/her heads. But I cannot say, "I hope everyone had a nice Thanksgiving Day and made time to reflect on all things in our lives that are important. We all have many things to be thankful for in our lives." It was a report on the November stroke newsletter. It took an hour for half the 14 people to share their lives. They have a lot to tell you, no doubt, but we have trouble attempting to speak. It could take 20 minutes individually about their hospitalization. People don't have the time!

It sounded a difficult vocation, working ones with aphasia. Volunteers Polly, Jan and Julie shared their moments. Imagine, at a meeting with patients, finding a string to an aphasic conversation? It should not be a meeting with volunteers or speech therapists. Anyone at the meeting should be an aphasic patient. If you're not a stroke survivor, then you are not expected to talk at the meeting. Orchestrating a conversation is ok. Maybe get a subject or a topic. Then, take a back seat. Aphasics (I can hardly speak it) should be at meetings. In other words, normal people are used to it. Are they're a metaphor: leader dogs to a blind man, or is the aphasic is the leader dog? Is there a translator who "talks" for stroke survivors?

Aphasia: a-fanta-sia. Fantasy is a daydream or really a nightmare, like the trilogy *Lord of the Rings*. A weird unearthly inhabited by hobbits written by J.R.R. Tolkien, but mostly orcs and demons and evil land of Mordor. "One Ring to rule them all, One Ring to find them. One Ring to bring them all and in the darkness bind them." Doesn't the voice bring us from a darkness that binds them? "In the Land of Mordor where the Shadows lie." As a fantasy world of unknown lands, willing to meet or unwilling to meet the world. To ignore what you speak and hear. Note that business (which all means "communication") is at our entire world. Are you going to be talking? Are you going to yell, "I want you to listen to my answer!"

"The Road goes ever on and on. Out from the door where it began. Now far ahead the Road has gone. Let others follow it who can!" said Tolkien. I was not handicapped so I would refuse to park for my car. I was NOT handicapped. But I WAS disabled. My vocal-machine was broken down.

Is disabled (crippled, halt, lame) leave me handicapped? I paid in a vacation to California for 35 cents for a trolley for disabled, which was $1. I wanted the driver to tell about my disabled, and my three months since a stroke, but he dismissed it. Every person expects the driver to sympathize all handicaps? Did I have a handicapped permit to earn me for 35 cents?

Handicapped is another word for renovated or universal design homes. They are accessible for all ages. Approximately 83% of people age 50 and older want to stay in their homes for the rest of their lives, according to a survey from American Association of Retired Persons (AARP). The design has a useful but appealing to all users, with a wide range of minimal hazards and accidents and an appropriate size if a space for each approach and use. Occupational therapists have literature obtaining mobility and convenience for their homes. Some contractors are familiar with the Americans with Disabilities Act Accessibility Guidelines (ADAAG) building or renovating designs. Remote or keyless entry is a boon to those in wheelchairs or walkers with people had a stroke. Bathrooms are standard seating in the tub or shower and grab bars on the bathtub walls. Kitchens can be lower cupboards or raising dishwashers so you load and unload dishes with a minimum amount of bending. There are also ramps, decks, wider doorways, open floor layouts, elevators, and so on. There's a tremendous need from the community for access to builders and universal design products that increase independence for handicapped persons. One builder is in my neighborhood, Arrow Building Co. of Sterling Heights, Mich. It built condominium units for Gateway Oaks in Sterling Heights, modifying a couple with removing a half-wall entry from the floor plan, and leaving a wide arch formed by a retaining post and a wall, for example. The kitchen leads to a mudroom, hallway and a garage door, were a ramp was built to give easy access. Grab bars were fitted to the wall next to the toilet and mounted on the wall on showers.

I had three daily medicines, only two drugs perscribed from one year after my stroke. From that day of the hospital I didn't before take medicines, even from vitamins. After my stroke, I took one 325 mg Bayer aspirin (capsule for coated time released), 100 mg Zoloft and 75 mg Plavix. All thin the blood. I really don't know whether I need these. I never needed any before. So why do I take them? Because of health insurance! I mean more correctly, defense or security. It's a warranty for your body. Like the ad says, "Plavix helps keep blood platelets from sticking together and forming cots, which helps protect you from another heart attack or stroke." As the strongest muscle in your body, your heart beats about 100,000 times and pumps 2,100 gallons of blood per day. I was thinking of taking one Bayer aspirin each Monday, one Tuesday to a Plavix, etc. Drugs were experimented with patients. Zoloft has been prescribed "are some symptoms of posttraumatic stress disorder... PTSD is a serious medical condition affecting over 13 million Americans." The cause is unknown, said Pfizer U.S. Pharmaceuticals. PTSD can be related to an imbalance of naturally occurring chemicals between nerve cells in the brain. A prescription drug works to correct this imbalance. Symptoms of depression vary from person to person. You may have five or more of the following symptoms and you have almost all of the time during the same two-week period. Changes in sleeping patterns; restlessness or slowed movements; fatigue or lack of energy; changes in appetite or weight; feeling worthless or guilty for no real reason; trouble concentrating or making decisions; repeated thoughts of death or suicide. Some people have a panic disorder and unexpected panic attacks. A panic attack is an unexpected attack of fear, anxiety or discomfort: fast heart rate or pounding heart; chest pain or discomfort; sweating; trembling or shaking; choking feeling; nausea or upset stomach; dizziness; etc.

I used to take all three drugs – Bayer, Plavix and Zoloft – taken in Thursdays, Fridays, Saturday and none on Sundays. (I have quit taking Zoloft. I had no depression or panic attacks.) This is post-stroke, sort of a menu, taking three drugs for six months, or two drugs for a year plus. After one year I am still taking Plavix and aspirin. Plavix is an ximelagatran, a blood thinner. The American Heart Association awarded one of the 10 top advances of 2003. After one year, I tried Aricept (5mg) every day. It's a drug for Alzheimer's disease that controls blood vessels flowing to the brain. Memantine is a similar drug for FDA approval to Alzheimer's, and has up to 40 experimental drugs. British researchers reported that Aricept had "disappointingly little overall benefit" and is not cost-effective. They said better treatments are needed. Most studies have shown that the drugs can produce small improvements in patients' scores on mental tests, but it is not clear whether those gains translate into anything helpful in real life. Experts in the United States already were divided over the usefulness of Aricept and related drugs and the study is unlikely to end the debate.

"Memory functions can be divided into three parts: registration, reinforcement and storage, and retrieval," according to Cleo Hutton and Louis Caplan, co-authors *of Striking Back At Stroke.* "To retain information, an individual must be attentive and interested in recalling the information and register it in the brain." Each sensation that enters the hippocampus, is a visual impression, setting off electrical charges inside the neurons. The charge stimulates the cell to release neurotransmitters, which carries information across gaps called synapses. A single neuron can have as many as 10,000, neurons retaining the data and the brain holds the storage or memory. It is important for memory if an individual is necessary for thinking and reasoning. In speech therapy, I tried to remember four or six words, or seven digits (it's integral to dial phone numbers). Four words unrelated from each other: suitcase, you, hair, mouth, for example. I can remember the words. Another sentence is more difficult for me. The pronouns were harder. I had an image in my mind with nouns and that was better: suitcase, hair and mouth. I didn't get a picture or image with pronouns: "you" or "he" or "mine". It was difficult for me so I concentrated with sentences and words. That was at a class from speech therapy 16 months prior my stroke.

I want to discuss my case for doctors, and quit my drugs (even aspirin), at least for a single day. I don't like taking drugs or medicine. I am a drug-free healthy human. But I had a stroke. Should I take a drug to thin my blood? Is it so important? Plavix, for one, is $20 or $30 for prescriptions, along with health insurance. That's easy, I'm told. Twenty bucks is cheap. Aspirin is even cheaper. That's not my point. My question: am I supposed to take my medicines daily? Every day, every week, every month? Is that so significant? Is my blood so important that drugs can dilute it?

'I guarantee it'

One thing I missed was reading, not just newspapers or magazines, but books or novels. After two years, I can read novels by John Grisham and Tom Clancy. But, after my stroke, it was really difficult to read these books. They were complex or complicated to me. They had too many pages and chapters. They were too difficult, too obscure, for me in the beginning, after the first year. At first, I tried a paperbook with word puzzles and jumbled letters: horizontal, vertical or diagonal. These puzzles were at least a book! Someone suggested to me after I had my stroke, an editor could play crosswords and word puzzles. I never liked crosswords and word puzzles. They were just a way of spending hours, I thought. But puzzles were honed my mind as my brain looks at words. They were a good example of learning words and learning to make sentences to make them longer or more comprehensible.

Words were words, words make sentences. Bed, lamp, and, make, cars, silverware, pretty. Words don't make sentences, usually. Soon after my stroke, words were unreadable. Newspapers and magazines have since become legible, after one month. I started out reading articles with its heading. Then with a single paragraph, then two paragraphs. I was ready with the public library. I always needed a fix, namely books. It was a comfortable rest for my evenings. I could take one book or two, for reading a new novel, maybe Frederick Forysth or Larry McMurtry, even if I couldn't read the entire book. Sometimes only a page, then 5 pages or 10 pages. Having that book in my hands is pleasurable to me. I yearn for reading. Accuracy is more important reading, then followed by speed. It was too hard when I was reading with distractions: watching t.v., hearing radios and listening voices. I could read, but didn't remember the pages. It was helpful if I had it quiet in my home. It was difficult reading with two teenagers in the house, talking the telephone, ringing the doorbell, etc. but it was easier if I had a quiet environment.

"Reading: for the books it is a source of pleasure, an opportunity to gain knowledge, or a way to spend hours enjoying the beauty of the printed word... No matter what the reading interest or need, most of us would find it devastating to be without this skill," wrote *Pathways, Moving Beyond Stroke and Aphasia*. Susan Adair Ewing and Beth Pfalgraf said: "Learning to read again following a stroke is not the same process as when we first acquired that skill... Given time and work, reading can become functional again." Now I have the time to relax reading books. And now, I have books that are difficult, too tedious for the level of 5th grade readers. There are stacks of books that are unread. I knew that. I'm still trying to read and re-read my appreciated authors and books.

At six months from my stroke, I read my first complete book. It was *I: The Creation of a Serial Killer* by Jack Olsen. It was at the new book section at the library. I thumbed it and looked it interesting and *all chapters were still two or three pages!* I could read every chapter after only one sitting. He was "the dean of true crime," according to the cover. Olsen is a journalist, like me. His wording was that of newspapers, and it gave the readers a reality. The nonfiction book was an interview and excerpts from the killer, a 6'6" truck driver who was a husband and a father of two children. He had a long-suffered, lost life – a story for my aphasia. I thought about my two years after my stroke. I remembered journalist Olsen's subject's life. Some things I had to re-read the second time. I had to reread certain paragraphs, but they were incomplete. Maybe I read a single sentence in the last paragraph, and it forced me to read the prior sentence or sometimes the second prior sentence. Maybe this sounds crazy, but it works! I had to re-sign it once at the library, so it took three weeks and another two weeks. Not good, not bad, for me. Olsen's book was 359 pages. I felt was a good reader. That's important for me, my lifetime and my career. My second and third books were on my next reading list. If they were not too difficult, and not too long, they were in my second reading list.

My second book post-stroke I read *Twelve* by Nick McDonnell, the writer who was born in 1984. I was 30 years old in 1984. He was 17 when he was an author! A book jacket was a recommendation for "Twelve" from writer and gonzo journalist Hunter S. Thompson, who is a favorite of mine. It's only for 244 pages, and for short chapters! Even better is a third book I also got from the public library. It's written by comedian Al Franken. I remembered him. I was covering contractors' roofing convention from a trade magazine, when I was a publisher and where he was a keynote speaker. Franken wrote his book, *Oh, the Things I Know!* It's a slim 153 pages and has even shorter chapters. I valued for humor during these blackest days in my life. The subtitle is "A Guide to Success, or, Failing That, Happiness." I replaced on the shelves a book called "The Forsyte Saga" by John Galsworthy. It was a bad time. Long chapters, and a full 878 pages. Maybe some day. Some books are too hard. I've tricked them, with a page and then re-reading it again; sometimes from the ending back to the beginning. It works. Books printed "LARGE PRINT" is also good, even if your eyes are a blessing. I enjoyed (Large Print) reading "Flyboys" by James Bradley after 1 ½ year after my stroke. It was "a true story of courage" in a historical book with World War II. I recommend the book, and also the large print (its 600-plus pages). His stories of brave men in the warplanes were unforgettable, a tragic epic of two empires in the Pacific Ocean. He shivered me with the words, "'I believe it was dark when a sailor brought in a package of something wrapped up in a newspaper,'" Yoshii's orderly, Suzuki, later testified. "The sailor told me it was sent by the captain and that I should keep custody of it. Therefore, I left it in the galley. Later on in the evening, the captain requested me to bring this package to him. Yoshii said, "Bring me the flesh which in your keeping." Suzuki unwrapped the package for Yoshii. 'It was a very dark-colored piece of flesh,' Suzuki said. 'I did not know whether liver looks like this, and I cannot say that it was liver.'" It was. It was about cannibalism. He told about, for one, man-eaters with Japan's soldiers (exactly with officers) during the war. And how America's Flyboys with their own B-29 Superfortresses launched Japan's people from firebombing and napalm during the last days of the war. It was heart-breaking and exhilarating but it calmed me with my personal, dreary, life. My life was insignificant with my stroke, if you read the words of Mr. Bradley.

After almost two years ago from the stroke, I read (large print) *The King of Torts*, by John Grisham. I liked it, but I was proud after I can read it too.

At first, friends said that I should read easy books, like teenage mysteries or novels, or even books by Dr. Seuss (author Theodor Geisel) or comic books (I liked Jughead and Green Lantern) or magazines like *Reader's Digest*. I read them all, and they read easier. Readers Digest challenged teenagers with college scholarships via its National Word Power Challenge. Maybe, but it wasn't the point. Reading was not simply the objective. I like reading, but I don't read for the books, the pages, and the words. I like reading for ideas or information or, at least, a thriller or a humorous book. That's why I read a lot. I like to read magazines, i.e. *National Geographic*, *Scientific American*, *Popular Science*, *Esquire*, and *Rolling Stone*, etc. It's harder for reading certain topics or authors, but it's exhilarating and stimulating for me. Reading is easier if you like or interested in their topics.

I write the words with my computer (Windows 95, then tried with Windows 98 and Word 6.0) and various HP and Lexmark printers. I long for a job. Work the words, I told my HP computer. After you've done it so many years, it can be easier for you. Just you are trying to type words, it can be the brain which speaks the throat. They're your brain doesn't hurt your hands. While the hurt or the sickness, your brain doesn't need no "hands," but needs your throat. My employer once asked if it took me a long time, pre-stroke. Sometimes I wrote an article, say five pages, only a few minutes. If I wanted to write, it was just the typing that took a time. Maybe 15 minutes, or a half-hour. Today, I write everything that have to be spoken out loud. Grab a dictionary. The thesaurus, too. It's grueling. I get the encyclopedia and *Bartlett's Famous Quotations* because I fail or can't explain or remember things that I have easily remembered then. At first I was typing, not writing. I typed my own articles. It's gibberish, to me. Jobberwocky. At first, I took the time, and it… slowly, sounded like some words familiar to me.

Too many aphasics make it too slow to speak. "Good........ morning....... for.........my .... friends." That isn't just a joke.

31

With aphasics take time for each or all of the words. Each word is succinct. Pronunciation is a foreign language.

Too many people will offer their words and not to hear them. They will shrug their shoulders and say, "I don't know what you want. If you can put it better so that I can understand it, or maybe write it." *Write it?* Oh well, give me a pen and paper and I will write it to you if you want. Is it really that simple? Writing is hard. Reading is hard. Speaking is hard after you have aphasia. From this moment, life has begun:

From this moment you are the one
Right beside you
is where I belong
From this moment on

From this moment I have been blessed
I live only for your happiness
And for your love I'd give my last breath
From this moment on

I give my hand to you with all my heart
Can't wait to live my life with you, can't wait to start
You and I will never be apart
My dreams came true because of you

From this moment as long as I live
I will love you, I promise you this
There is nothing I wouldn't give
From this moment on

You're the reason I believe in love
And you're the answer to my prayers from up above
All we need is just the two of us
My dreams came true because of you
(Anonymous)

Editing your sentences

"I..... want...... to....."

"You want to walk a nice place in outdoors? Sure, let's go!"

They mentioned something like " want to drive my car to the store." This might be the right sentence. If people are willing to wait for the longer sentence, they will learn and communicate to me. My sentences in therapy classes are: The hunter _____ (shot) the duck. I will _____ (clips) these papers together. The _____ (paper) was full of ads. Two people were _____ (shot) in the holdup.

For my classes in December 2002 speech therapy, it sounded like baby steps. I saw the questions: *1) clip 2) paper 3) shot.* Two people were shot in the holdup. I tried at synonyms: parts of a car. Engine, transmission, radiator, power steering pump, fan, mirrors, doors, wiper blades. I did four or five words to think a sentence: find, can't, my, sweater, I. I can't find my sweater. The finished of a sentence: the 6:00 news. What now is on television? Give a word with six *sh* starts. Shadow, share, shatter, sheer, she, shit (give the therapist a laugh). Add the words: roller (coaster); french-fried (potatoes), snow (blizzard). Circles the ones that are spelled incorrectly: scissors, thyme, excercise, which, importent, direct. They are exercise and important. It's easy. But does it make me learn sentences? Does it loop paragraphs, more to make them two or three together? Does it make me better at copy editing, or a managing editor? Therapy doesn't make me a job (especially publisher). Only a copy editing test would take that. They would have to give me a "real" job. My therapist told me, "You have a plateau." I've gotten as far as I can. I hated her conclusion. It means, as she calls it, nearer to my therapy, not a concrete wall inside my maze. My class may mean the objective. It may be to thread more sentences, and then thread into paragraphs, so it could be conversations. I hope so. The English language sounds so familiar and, then again, it's unfamiliar and foreign. Take five or six words in a thesaurus that still makes another word. But a word sounds "special" and you think everything makes sense. I told my neighbor, a teacher, because she got a sore throat and she should take an excuse for her day. She needed a sick-day. I told her that I'd write her a "message" to excuse for her classes. "Message" doesn't really mean to communicate. It's the word "note" that I wanted to write for her excuse. I emailed with another friend. I wrote: You cleaned your car? I meant: You washed your car? It's the same, but sounds a little better after the second sentence.

It's too many words for typos. An editor would cringe at so many typos.

Speak one word that gives me a guess, a notion. "Restaurant" means a defined noun that differs from my "house" or the "store." A common noun modifies a definite noun. "Jovan's Restaurant" tells them a certain, common place a mile from my house, on a street on Dodge Park. It tells me its meaning, its place, it tells me everything. We have eaten before. Just the two words, it tells me a lot. But when I say, "Let's go to dinner at Jovan's Restaurant, we'll eat later at 7 p.m." it can be a mouthful. What about Jovan's Restaurant? What do you want to go to dinner, and what time? They might need directions. You're up to 12 words, perhaps more! A sentence that it assumes a conversation. Two words mean a simpler statement, and then a question.

Chapter 3

It's not an illness

Broca's aphasia is not an illness. Nor is it a handicap. It's a road that means to communicate. The way to read, and write, and speak by learning communication by understanding English. You learn to what you have first learned at the age of 3 or 4. I am a child.

Aphasia is being a thorough subject for reading. Not like I'm an aphasia phobic, you see. But it takes a lot of time, study, and my life. On the book, *Men's Health for Dummies*, there is seven pages on strokes: ischemic (one blood vessel blocked) by and hemorrhagic (caused by a head injury caused by a hematoma, or pooled blood). It was valuable, but skim and skinny. It has a chapter, "Surgery: Is It Really Necessary?" There are 21 pages about cancer, and explanations of heartburn or nail fungus. It was seven pages on losing your hair (hair loss information in www.hairloss.com). The sexual development, contraceptives and three more chapters on sexually transmitted diseases and condoms all finish at 51 pages. Aphasia didn't even make the index, or the chapter on stroke. The reality is that his penis is more important than his brain!

Although it's a sensitive to talk with others, coping with intimacy and sex after a stroke can play a key role. The closeness that a couple shares affects how their relationship afterwards. It's necessary for couples to experience a sense of loss whenever one has a stroke. Studies show that sex plays a significant role in our self-esteem and emotional well-being. It's central to our lives. We think about sex once a day for 54% men and 19% women, according to a study. No two people are exactly the same in their level of interest. Because of this variability, there really is no such thing as a normal frequency. Intimacy becomes more important with age.

"The landmark of sensory aphasia, later to become Wernicke's aphasis, was thus described by Wernicke as the sutult of a lesion in the dominant first temporal gyrus. The area first postulated by Meynert and subsequently named Wernicke's area for its descriptor. The primary deficit sensory aphasia, according to Wernicke was an interruption of the central auditory projection area, or klagfeld (soundfeld.)" *Aphasia and Related Neurogenic Language Disorders,* a textbook on the current therapy of communication disorders, with series editor William Perkins, is sometimes hard to understand. But understanding is the message. "The resultant dysprosody is characterized by a slowly speech rate, inappropriate stress patterns, pauses between syllables, a marked interruption of the inflectional contour and reduced loudness."

Less than three hours have to help a patient's condition. A CT (computerized axial tomography) angiography can look any blood vessels that are restricted or restrained. This will find an aneurysm under a CT scan it can track blood as it leaves the brain. Eighty-five percent of all strokes can be treated using either blood clotting drugs or operations through an artery or a blood vessel via a groin or leg. A heart surgery to an aneurysm can be a critical operation to the patients. My first and last operation was searching for the heart from my right thigh. It's routine in a heart operation. It's safer than open heart surgery. The forceps found my heart, starting from my inner thigh. It lasted an hour. The operation was almost 30 days after my stroke. One day from Saturday and one day exempt from running, on Sunday. After Monday I was running, with the bluish mark of the blood vessel in the thigh leaving the only souvenir of my operation. (My thigh had a yucky bluish look, like blueberry pies.)

Another patient, 30, had a stroke. He had a dilemma, with no risk factors and no family history of stroke. He had a hole in his heart, like mine. Said one doctor, "If someone has a stroke at a young age, that is often an indication of a hole in the heart." Almost 25% of all people had a hole in their hearts that are unnoticed, like me. Strokes allow blood clots to flow through the heart into the bloodstream. At once, treating holes in the heart required open-heart surgery. Not anymore. A catheter is in the groin or thighs and through the veins until it reaches the heart. An echocardiogram and angiogram are allowed him to view the heart and measure the size of the hole.

A therapist from St. John Hospital said, "Aphasia is not a goal" and it's a speech-language disorder. Aphasia is the difficulty with:

1) Comprehension
2) Verbal speech
3) Reading
4) Writing

"Generalization of improved lexical retrieval beyond the production of single words should also be sought," the textbook pinpoints the topic. "Generally, speakers are asked to produce successively longer utterances beginning with two-word combinations and gradually increasing the length of their utterances depending on their success at previous levels."

Some of these things surprised me:

In my mind I was a little wary, long after two years that my voice would disappear or fade. I feel like I was going to speak from my voice box and the voice box would go silent if I couldn't use it.

I had to relearn a computer. Gateway was in my workplace vs. a Hewlett Packard in my office-home. It was much of a big surprise, because minor differences with hardware, software, Internet, emails, and printer, confused me. I had to study with my computer, going back to bookshelves with manuals and reading about Windows95, Windows ME, XP, Office, Excel, 98, etc. At once it was people who fiddled our machines and our software. I really needed them and wanted them! I was anxious and angry because little problems stopped my writing.

Taking new university speech pathology classes: I thought from the comedian Rodney Dangerfield in his "Spring Break" movie. I was taking in classes with age 48. When I asked my therapist, "There are co-eds in classes?" When asked if I enrolled a speech pathology class, I said, with wry comment, "Yes, I'm teaching a class."

My therapists and instructors said that my "youthful" (48) was among the stroke patients. "He's so young," said the veteran patient. They were in the 60s and 70s. Most patients had grandchildren. Plenty of survivors had strokes in the ages of 30s and 40s. .

"Your company has been much harder to get your job that you are disabled," someone told me. It's true. After two years, I am disabled. What job is that? I can type. You can teach chimpanzees to type words, if you have the time. What does the word "disabled" mean? Sometimes, disabled can link hands with brain, and brain with mouth. They seem like I am rested on the bench, getting better, stronger, "abled." After six months, from a year, from two years. A year is an eternal. But really it is not. I was 48. I am 50-plus when I'll be ready to work. I am better, stronger, and healthier. I am still disabled, too. If you're an employer, would you give me a job... age 50, had a stroke, aphasia, disabled, a handicap?

Tennis is a good, quick game for me. My son, Derek, a few weeks after my stroke, finished my tennis sets at 6-1, 6-2. But what or how or why my tennis stroke terminated from my stroke? Was my eyes or my footsteps, there a little miscued from I left in the hospital? Or was Derek better at this season, this year (he was also 19)? Or was it my getting older, my eyes were bad and my nerves or stamina got a little worse? Was I too slow from brain-eyes-hands-legs to chase a tennis ball? Maybe I was slower, that's all. An old fart.

I write about a side incident about St. John Hospital. It's nothing, the incident itself, but it tells a lot. I registered to the hospital at Saturday for my original stroke. I came to conscious on Sunday, ate a lot, slept, I had a relaxed walk on Wednesday. An outside "relaxed" walk to five or six miles to my house. This was a little scary, I was told. But not to me. It was the fourth day of sitting and lying in bed. I was bored. The hospital was bored, too. Four days recently was a stroke but seeming like it was months ago. My intravenous with rubber tubing was carefully put on a night side table. My shoes were under the bed. I was wearing shorts and a t-shirt. I nonchalantly walked to the elevator, although I was staring at people. No one did. There was no anxiety. Again, the first time, I felt a free prisoner! The lobby was no difference to my first glance. The outside it was warm, the sunny was early afternoon. I looked to south, not at first knowing the directions, and the first street was guessed at Hoover. Hoover didn't go to the main street, Dodge Park. It was three miles or so but I took one street that was a dead end. To my house, I walked west one mile, north one mile and one east. It was a long way! It took me almost two hours, which was about five or six miles.

The day was still nice. Warm, not hot. Six miles was not too much, I once ran five miles, maybe six or seven. But this takes me a lot of time as walking. The hospital wanted to see me. My family was so concerned *after the patient was lost.* I was almost six miles when I was walked from two blocks of my house. It was my wife and daughter, Kathy and Shannon who saw me, from their car. It was my ex-wife who turned away on my beeline at the hospital! I was almost home. I regretted it. For some really good food, eight hours of sleep, and not any nurses or aids awaking me in my hospital ward. The clock was ticking. My hours and days cost me, financially, from the doctor bills, specialists, tests, and hospitalization partly from health insurance. Don't think you'll be safer from the hospital's bills. Insurance usually picks up 80%. If your hospital costs $100,000, your bill will cost you $20,000. That's a huge problem.

It wasn't a big deal, my walking to my home four days after my stroke. Some stroke survivors, like Marc Hardin, a 51-year-old veterinarian, has almost 70 marathons, one of them a marathon six months after he had his stroke. One 35-year-old man ran a half-marathon and played golf, bowling and racquetball. Good luck! I really mean that. I can do the same things, fortunately. I run, bicycle, bowling, golf, tennis, volleyball – there is almost I can play without speaking ("That's a damn stinky shot," I often mumbled.)

I could find my voice box but there was something dreadfully wrong. But it's not a big deal. It's not that I was Frank Albert Sinatra (or even Tom Waits). If I wanted to yell, or scream "Help!" or

"Watch you're driving, dumb ass," I could have made a sound. The miles at home made me a little thirsty, but there was no problem. I was 100% conscious, with all the faculties and capacity. I was awake, not sleeping, though sometimes they said I was a moron – or at least a little foolish six miles walking to my home.

I was admitted once again into the hospital. I was with a nursing student via a bodyguard, 24 hours every day. I feel they were guarding Marlon Brando in the Godfather. Bodyguards didn't help him, did they? Those working at bodyguards at St. John Hospital were pleasant, others were dozing asleep. I could feel their pain! I was no fun. I slept, watched t.v., ate. I didn't attempt to escape again, although they'd secure my shoes. I'll spend the hospital at least six days again from my initial four days: 10 days altogether. It was lethally boring. Testing in the hospital rooms, tests and tests. There was nothing to see, nothing to do. They would look into my brain and find…nothing! It was competent, normal food. Nothing bad, except avoiding a salt shaker. I could walk faster than my physical therapy instructor. I had a lot of walking, from the hallway before the elevators until my room. Six days before I was ready. But I didn't have my voice from my voice box. I went from the hospital 10 days without my speech. From six months ago from my stroke, adding three times for weekly per speech therapy, it did not help my voice. I left it at St. John Hospital. I left at meetings, classes, seminars, etc. to find my voice. My voice was not easy. It was elusive. How hard and difficult but so simple was my voice?

Two days after my 10 days in the hospital, I returned to my work. The boss was dumbfounded! Here I was, 12 days from my stroke, at my office, at my desk. There was two weeks, or nine weekdays. I was afraid losing my vacation days and was reluctant my sick days were gone, too. My boss came to me at my desk to shake my hand, and said something like, "I didn't think you were here so quickly." I was unwilling to go home when I wasn't really sick. I didn't have the flu, wasn't feverish or having headaches or nausea. I took only a few days in working over 10 years. I felt fine. Two weeks was, well, that was two whole weeks of excuses. After I drove this morning with my van at exactly eight miles. I was going to open my mail, see the emails on my computer, and maybe see if someone had called me. That was a routine day. I knew that wasn't a lot of work. In my magazine, I tried to type an article for a preceding issue. It was a struggle. The words didn't give me the right information. They were gibberish. Still, emails were just enough to understand or readable. They are written in a minute. I loved the emails. No one worried about spelling or punctuation or grammar. I am starting to shorten my sentences. Two, three, or even five or six or seven words. That's good! Sometimes writers keep a sentence to 20 or even 27 or even 32 words, and that's a good thing, some writers said. I thought it's a bad idea. How many words have you written in your sentences? Seven or eight? Two? You've lost the readers at words number 20 or number 30. My pre-stroke article was the subject of an interview. My article began: "Mike Palazzolo changed." Who is he? Why did he change? He was a contractor and he had a good job, a good life. A reporter shortens his or her lead.

Six months after my stroke, I wondered if I should give up my career? After almost 30 years a journalist, I could type, reading and editing. Should I get a job, one without phoning or interviewing, or even talking?

My boss and employees weren't too keen to keep on my job. They were thinking that I wasn't "all right". Your communication (and *not* communication) deals a lot. "Are you ok?" A smile, "Uh-huh." It wasn't satisfactory to my condition, and to my improvement. They phoned my sister to take me at my home. It was the last straw. I was thrown out. Kindly, and fairer. Go get better. *Please!* My van was in the parking lot. How was I going to get it at home? I told that I could drive it. So many drunks are held back for the keys. I wasn't drunk. I didn't have any driving failures, dizzy spells or unconsciousness. "I can drive," I said. I drove the full eight miles. Why not? Was there a crash or an accident to occur? I drove for another six months without an accident or without a ticket. A year plus, now. I cannot imagine with my driver's license. I cherish my precious driver's license. I'd be able to drive my car when I was able to drive, from therapy to stores, to send my daughter Shannon to school. A year from my stroke, I had a chauffeur's operator license in case of getting a driving job – temporarily – in lieu of a writer.

My ex-wife and son were reluctant to give me the keys. I used a substitute, "secret" ignition key that was hidden under my rear bumper. The key was put in there a year ago to unlock the car in case I lost my original key. I got my keys, my car, and my freedom.

My trade magazine takes me writing to another industry: hvac, or heating, ventilation and air conditioning. Along with indoor air quality and mold, the current news, along with insurance, marketing, advertising, web sites, tools, retiring, buying and selling your business, hires and fires, the newest trucks, gadgets and trade ideas. It's a gigantic world, tens of thousands of readers. Many conventions and conferences are held by sheet metal contractors, building engineers, maintenance and facilities, hvac and service contractors, etc. in Las Vegas, Orlando, Chicago, San Francisco, Dallas, Boston, Hawaii. The medical industry has its own meetings and conventions. For stroke meetings was convened by the American Heart Association and National Stroke Association. Medical personnel have a meeting to spread news and tidbits for patients. Join us for the American Heart Association's Scientific Sessions, they told us – "the world's largest convention for scientists and healthcare professionals devoted to the science of cardiovascular disease and stroke."

A division of the American Stroke Association, part of American Heart Association held by a national meeting for aphasia. They said that more than 3,700 presentations given by "experts" in the areas of cardiovascular disease. They feature "current advances" (not old-fashioned advances) which are, for example, surgery, cerebral circulation, brain function, clinical stroke research and rehabilitation. Spend time in the growing exhibit hall. They feature state-of-the-art stroke related equipment and services (again, publicity: maybe better than old-timer equipment). State-of-the-art, advanced, current, high-tech... you get the message. Exhibitors will hold a menu at a trade meeting, of equipment from stroke survivors: from doctors to diagnostics, and research to insurance. Don't forget Bristol-Myers Squibb/Sanofi Pharmaceuticals (makers of Plavix, the anticoagulant clopidogrel bisulfate). Bristol-Myers and Pfizer together produce 12 of the 25 top-selling drugs in 2004. Aggrenox is a key player in a clinic trial, along with Exanta (ximelagatran) made by AstraZeneca. Either one is an effect with warfarin, an anticoagulant drug. Either one prevent blood platelets from sticking together to form clots that would restrict blood flow. The only difference is they affect the platelets. The risk of recurrent stroke in patients who have had a first stroke is significant due to degenerative processes in the wall of blood vessels. The stroke risk ranges from 3-10% in the first month, 5-15% within a year, and 25-40% within five years. Warfarin is the only alternative for almost 50 years. It's necessary to monitor for dose adjustment and interacts with some foods and drugs.

A coordination of strokes

The National Stroke Association was held a North American stroke convention in December 4-6, 2003 in Orlando, Fla. It held the 5th annual World Stroke Congress in June 23-26, 2004, in Vancouver, B.C., Canada. The National Aphasia Association was in June 3-6 in Tampa, Fla. and cosponsored by the University of South Florida. Is aphasia-friendly different to best practice guidelines for general readability? Do people with aphasia receive information while they are in hospital?

The brain is divided into four primary parts: the right hemisphere (or half), the left hemisphere, the cerebellum and the brain stem. The right hemisphere of the brain controls the movement of the left side of the body. It also controls analytical and perceptual tasks, such as judging distance, size, speed, or position and seeing how parts are connected to wholes. A stroke in the right hemisphere often causes paralysis in the left side of the body. This is known as left hemiplegia. Survivors of right-hemisphere strokes may also have problems with their spatial and perceptual abilities. This may cause them to misjudge distances (leading to a fall) or be unable to guide their hands to pick up an object, button a shirt or tie their shoes. They may even be unable to tell right-side up from upside-down when trying to read. Along with their impaired ability to judge spatial relationships, survivors of right-hemisphere strokes often have judgment difficulties that show up in their behavioral styles. These patients often develop an impulsive style unaware of their impairments and certain of their ability to perform the same tasks as before the stroke. This behavioral style can be extremely dangerous. It may lead the left hemiplegic stroke survivor to try to walk without aid. Or it may lead the survivor with spatial and perceptual impairments in attempt to drive a car (like me).

Survivors of right-hemisphere strokes may also experience left-sided neglect. Stemming from visual field impairments, left-sided neglect causes the survivor of a right-hemisphere stroke to "forget" or "ignore" objects or people on their left side. Finally, some survivors of right-hemisphere strokes will experience problems with short-term memory. Although they may be able to recount a visit to the seashore that took place 30 years ago, they may be unable to remember what they ate for breakfast that morning.

The left hemisphere of the brain controls the movement of the right side of the body. It also controls speech and language abilities. A left-hemisphere stroke often causes paralysis of the right side of the body. This is known as right hemiplegia. A second danger is that increased blood pressure can burst an artery or push a blood clot into a smaller vessel, also called a thrombus. Similarly, an embolus is the mass of foreign material. If the rupture, embolus or thrombus, deprives tissue of blood supply, it will die. The tissue is a condition called a cerebrovascular accident, or a stroke. Ray Bradbury, author of "The Martian Chronicles" and "The Illustrated Man," had a stroke at the age of 83. He rarely made trips to his library anymore, with books scattered in his house in southern California. Roy Horn (the entertainer with Siegfried and Roy) also had a stroke after an attack by a tiger in a Las Vegas show.

Someone who had a left-hemisphere stroke may also have a case of aphasia. Aphasia is a catch-all term used to describe a wide range of speech and language problems. These problems can be highly specific, affecting only one component of the patient's ability to communicate, such as the ability to move their speech-related muscles to talk properly. The same patient may be completely unimpaired when it comes to writing, reading or understanding speech. In contrast to survivors of right-hemisphere stroke, patients who had a left-hemisphere stroke often develop a slow and cautious behavioral style. They need frequent instruction and feedback to complete tasks.

Finally, patients with left-hemisphere stroke may develop memory problems similar to those of right-hemisphere stroke survivors. These problems can include shortened retention spans, difficulty in learning new information and problems in conceptualizing and generalizing. The cerebellum controls many of our reflexes and much of our balance and coordination. A stroke that takes place in the cerebellum can cause abnormal reflexes of the head and torso, coordination and balance problems, dizziness, nausea and vomiting.

Strokes that occur in the brain stem are especially devastating. The brain stem is the area of the brain that controls all of our involuntary, "life-support" functions, such as breathing rate, blood pressure and heartbeat. The brain stem also controls abilities such as eye movements, hearing, speech and swallowing. Since impulses generated in the brain's hemispheres must travel through the brain stem on their way to the arms and legs, patients with a brain stem stroke may also develop paralysis in one or both sides of the body.

Chapter 4

A better and healthy student

While I am waiting, I will be a better and healthier student. But I was eager for my goal: in my three months, I was going to a job, as an editor and publisher. Three months and the goal is a distant one. (My goal was after one year getting a job with an editor and publisher. My goal was after two years getting a job, etc.) My speech therapist, Amy, asked, "If you are there yet?" I wasn't there. No, it was just a goal. The goal was a rubbery, inconstant, variable goal. Amy said that three months was a little time. I made my new(er) goal. It made for four months (30 days for speech therapy!) to be able to work. The goal is not a deadline, nor a dead end. My newest goal is six months from my original goal. Six months to get a job. Six months to communicate. Six months to say to a woman and invite her out to dinner in a restaurant. Or to dance or seeing a movie with a date. SIX MONTHS! I said. It doesn't work. The definition for goal is "aim" or "purpose," not the ending or the objective.

After three months, its goal was in October 2002. In November it was four months, and six months from January 2003. My Wayne State University speech therapy classes began in January 22, 2003, in a university campus in Detroit. Rehabilitation meetings at St. John Hospital North Shores include outpatients around the same month. I take to attend just to talk to someone, somewhere. Patients in a meeting who are learning to read, write, and speak. The walls at my house don't talk to me. Where do you take time for a full time job and a full time class? No problem. With two years after my stroke, I probably am ready for a job. But not as a publisher, not as an editor. My company doesn't need me. That's good! I was a player with a team. The same mind is okay. The same brain almost will handle it, I ask for it. Except for conversations. I read on a stroke magazine that six months after a left side of brain houses all the language. At this time, the right brain believes its left side is *broken*. It's time to learning and try a right hand (or right brain) to learn the language. Researchers at Washington University School of Medicine in St. Louis, Mo., have demonstrated that when the language areas of the left side of the brain are injured by a stroke, the right side can take over. It will learn to perform language. Neurons can be helped to grow in the brains. Dirt, seeds, water, plants, sunshine, minerals... composting them, a gardener can do it! The problem is no really knows which the neurons have language or movement. Another one is an antibody that can clear blockheads in blood as a plaque. Just how antibodies remove plaques remains unknown. A problem is the antibodies are typically too large to cross the blood-brain barrier. Another one, linoleic acid, can somewhat reduce stroke. It can decrease blood pressure and reduce the blood from clotting. Linoleic acid is found in corn, sunflower and soybeans.

I spend two hours a day at writing my books and articles. Then I worked an hour at Internet reading at USA Today and Detroit Free Press, etc. 1stheadlines.com offers current headlines with links to a full article from 300-plus newspapers and broadcasts. The problem with other ways of learning the Internet for people with aphasia are texts are still too complex, classes are intimidating, too fast and do not offer much individual help. You need basic computer skills for on-line tutorials. I talk to friends or employers-employees, editors and writers, to their emails. Then one hour at reading books. Something good, something less-than-good. Or going to the public library. Books, magazines, videos and videocassettes (like the Healing Arts: Communication with a topic of aphasia and Time Life Medical with the helpful Stroke: at Time of Diagnosis). After, I will take two hours at the exercise at the YMCA or outdoors at running in the park or subdivisions, and two hours take me at grocery stores and always various errands. The time runs out in a day, and I feel like I am working.

It's hard for me to take away two words: running and writing. One takes me for the other. Running makes my brain working and my writing makes me run.

"Hello, I have a left brain that doesn't seem to work."

"Dis is Stan. Come again?"

"I have a left brain. It doesn't work. The right one seems to work all right. It's the communication and it's troublesome. I wonder if it will start out with the right brain, or would I have a left one to speak steady? You got one from the shelves? Or maybe you can fix the one that I have, although it's only 49 years old?"

"Uhhhh... this is a muffler service. You want a muffler for your car?"

"You know that in England you drive the opposite of your streets. I feel that if you can drive in England, it's appropriate and proper legal. Sort of like driving with a right brain, even though your left brain isn't working right."

"Uh, what kind of car is that?"

"Not a car. Not a truck. It's known as aphasia. A disorder that results from damage to language centers of the brain. I've had it for a year from my stroke. A long time. Getting too long, getting it a long time, you understand?"

"Dis is Stan. Ya say you wanna muffler?"

The brain is a mass of pink-gray tissue within the cranium. It weighs about three pounds. It consists of the cerebrum, the cerebellum, the medulla oblongata and the pons varolii. The cerebrum is the language center. They are connected to the body with a spinal cord and vertebrae. These are the nerve fibers. There are many ways of a brain with its signals to the body, of course, the brain tumor and stroke. The functional unit of the nervous system is the nerve cell, or neuron. The neuron keeps the proton and the electron in the atoms – NOPE! Keep awake, I am losing you. Motor nerves will transmit impulses from the brain and spinal cord to the muscles.

Mixed nerves have motor and sensory fibers, and are capable of moving messages, just as an email for its software and computer.

The signs of stroke: You're at least someone understands. "This is important for your survival as well as theirs." I didn't have any warning signs of a stroke. Sudden numbness or weakness of the face, arm or leg, especially on one side of the body. Sudden confusion had also trouble speaking. There was trouble, seeing in one or both eyes. Trouble for walking, dizziness, balance loss or coordination. I didn't see it. Not for a single moment, or any symptoms.

About my friend, Craig, tells me about the left side and the right side. He is fairly smart. He is retired from a telecommunications expert. "Our brains have always been broken," he emailed. "Ever since Ruddiman (eighth year junior high, which we graduated). Nowadays, it's just that someone else tells us so. To hell with them. Our brains just work differently at this time." I thought about it. He was right.

Writing for disabilities

It's time for me to write people with their disabilities. Fifty-four million have Americans have the subject of disability. I learn them everyday. I'm disabled, and a writer. Don't make them disabled, don't term them disabled, if they aren't. Use regular instead of normal when referring to people. Take to consider these steps:

- Write, "He/she is a wheelchair user," rather than "He/she is confined to a wheelchair."
- Avoid using handicapped to describe people.
- Don't mention a disability if it's not relevant to the article (the driver is disabled though he wasn't ticketed or had an accident by a police report).
- Avoid words promoting stereotypes like crippled, lame, retarded, crazy, spastic and stupid.
- Use regular instead of normal when referring to people. What is "normal?"

Many stroke survivors can read aids on training, exercise and rehabilitation. Traditional arm slings are complicated and difficult to use. Some complain of neck and shoulder pain from wearing slings. Training for our arms allows using their arms and hands for grasp and releases. They'll read about free prescriptions or large type editions for books and magazines (they are available from public libraries). They want to get information on diets; i.e. the potassium (bananas and apples) and milk of magnesium (they can soothe people from cramps.) Readers and aphasia conversion will learn to help the paperback, for example, the "21st Century Synonym and Antonym Finder" and electronic mini- and pocket-PCs. They can hold entire dictionaries and thesauruses, and is easier.

From my aphasic meetings, we give success for each other. We yell and clap for when a silent mum tells us that it's his/her birthday! We play Scrabble, Boggle, Trivial Pursuit and other word-games, with synonyms that give our words when our right brain uses them. When someone gives a word, or a sentence, we give them an appreciative breakthrough. We told that all of the members at a meeting news about their grandson, or a grandniece, or the jobs we had once before retiring. At meetings, we read the newspapers (if only the headlines), books (if we can), crosswords, jigsaw puzzles and word seeking puzzles. Already, for the right side brain is going to, one day, speak out. Every single gets to him/her a turn. We're listening, even if they're quiet. Your time! Take your time, and say something, even a murmur or a nod or a whispering. Listen to his wife, or a son, or a daughter at their birthdays, a trip to the casinos with the senior citizens riding on a bus. Anybody, anything else to say?

The day was still nice in July when I was hospitalized. It was sunny and 80 degrees. It was really glorious! Six miles was not too much to walk, I ran once five miles, maybe six or seven. I ran the Bobby Crim for international top runners for 10 miles in Flint, Michigan. I ran it for 10 years annually. The Crim's premier event is a favorite of runners from across the globe every year around August 23. A 100-foot elevation after Bradley Hills added to the challenge of this scenic yet demanding course. High school bands, older people from the front yards with coffee, water stations every mile, etc. But it takes me a lot of walking. The hospital personnel wanted to see me. My family was so concerned. I was almost six miles after the hospital when I was only two blocks from my house. It was my wife and daughter who saw me, looking for me from their car. And it was my ex-wife who turned away on my beeline at the hospital! I was almost home.

It didn't surprise me after walking miles that day. What surprised me was that I couldn't find my voice box. I knew I had it, but it wasn't working. There was something wrong. But no such a big need. If I wanted to yell, or scream "help!" or "Watch you're driving, dumb ass." I could have made a sound. The miles at home made me a little thirsty, but there was no problem. I was 100% conscious, with all the faculties and capacity. I was awake, though sometimes they said I was a moron – or at least a fool.

I was turned again to the hospital. I was with a nursing student via a bodyguard, 24 hours a day. A nanny, better than a bodyguard. Some were pleasant, others were asleep. I could feel their pain! I was no fun. I didn't attempt to escape again, although they'd keep my shoes. I'll send at least six days in the hospital, 10 days altogether. It was crashing boring! Going to tests, tests and tests. There was nothing to see. Like the joke, it would look into my head and found nothing – no brains! Six days before I was ready. Good food. Nothing bad, except for deleting a salt shaker. And I could walk faster than the physical therapy instructor. But I didn't have my voice box. I gave the hospital 10 days without speaking. Six months ago, adding to three times per therapy, but did not help my voice. I left my words and my sentences at St. John Hospital.

He wasn't too keen

No one was the only one to see me. Two days after my 10 days in the hospital, I returned to my work. The boss was dumbfounded! Here I was, 12 days my stroke. There was two weeks, nine weekdays.

My boss came to me to shake my hand, and said something like "I didn't think you were that quick." I was reluctant to home when I was sick. I took only a few days in over 10 years. I felt fine. Two weeks was, well, that was two whole weeks of job time. After I drove eight miles this morning, I was going to open my mail, see the emails, and maybe see if someone had called me. I knew that wasn't a lot of work. In my magazine, I tried to type them. It was a struggle. The words didn't give me the right of information. They were almost unintelligible chatter. Emails were just enough to understand the words or sentences. I liked my emails. The emails replaced my spoken words.

But my boss and employees weren't too keen on my job. They were that I wasn't all right. Your communication deals a lot. "Are you ok?" A smile, "Uh-huh." It wasn't satisfactory to my improvement. They phoned my sister to take me at my home. It was the last straw. I was being thrown out. Kindly, and fair. Go get better. My car was in the parking lot. How was I going to get it at home? I told that I could drive it. So many drunks are held back for the keys. I wasn't drunk. I didn't have any driving failures, dizzy spells or unconsciousness. After acknowledgment, I drove eight miles. Why not? I drove for another six months without an accident or without a ticket. I cannot imagine with my driver's license. I'd be able to drive my car when I was able to drive, from therapy to store to send my daughter Shannon to school.

Diagnosing stroke

To determine whether symptoms are caused by a stroke, doctors may consider the following:
- A physical examination.
- Special tests of the nerves and reflexes.
- Laboratory analysis of samples of blood, urine or spinal fluid.
- An electrocardiogram (EKG or ECG), which can reveal heart problems.
- Scanning tests, such as computed tomography (CT) or magnetic

resonance imaging (MRI), that can reveal details of the brain's structure.

Private testing will perform a number of health disease, and stroke, some with a fee. It's sort of like glaucoma testing and blood pressure. Advanced Screening, of Grand Blanc, Michigan, and Life Line Screening of Cleveland, Ohio, are only a couple of private companies who perform risk factors in men and women who have previous strokes or transient ischemic strokes (TIA) or known as mini-strokes. Up to 40% of patients with mini strokes have silent heart disease. They have symptoms for high blood pressure; irregular heartbeat; heart disease; high blood cholesterol levels; smoking or heavy alcohol use; diabetes; advancing age; and family history of stroke or heart disease. Those with diabetes and high blood pressure (hypertension) dramatically raise the risk of "silent strokes." The screening companies have the equipment at the local YMCA, at the public libraries, senior citizen meetings, public health clinics and others.

For generations the American healthcare system has focused on disease management in a "crisis" mode, awaiting symptoms to appear prior to the intervention of physicians and medical professionals. However, it is commonly known that disease is a six-stage process. The first stage is being at risk. It is not until the fourth stage of disease that symptoms present themselves and the sixth stage is death. The form of screens and tests that concentrate on stages two and three where detection can have positive effects on the person's outcome. Without fasting, "yucky" liquids and laxatives, the ultrasound painless instrument will be moved around your neck to visualize the inside of the carotid artery. In a large room or auditorium, the companies have an advantage: no appointments, no individual rooms, no doctors there at the clinic or office. They can charge less than a test by the doctor. This can scan in the neck for plaque buildup. The #1 cause of stroke is linked to carotid artery blockage. Also, there are tests that have abdominal aortic aneurysm screening, peripheral arterial disease screening and osteoporosis screening (the bone density of the heel is measured with ultrasound).

A registered vascular technologist (RVT) and licensed practical nurse with fifteen years of experience in vascular ultrasound. A medical doctor does, finally, observe and analyze the tests. Dozens of aneurysms have been found through its work sites. Some have led to medical intervention while others are carefully being watched to monitor the disease progression. Knowledge of potential life threatening situations is invaluable knowledge to patients, health care professionals and doctors as well. With the addition of its heart screen (more commonly called echo) will be adding EKG and Hemoglobin A1C for three months glucose monitoring.

The CT scan at that time showed left middle cerebellar artery distribution attenuation defect consistent with a cerebral infarction. There was also persistent mass-effect in the left frontal horn of the ventricles, according to a doctor. My lesion suggested a left middle cerebral artery distributed a cerebrovascular problem. I had a cerebrovascular accident was in progression, said the report. There was a small to moderate right to left shunt through a patent foremen ovale. There was also a small atrial septal aneurysm. Said one doctor, I was recommended to have correction of this patent foramen ovale while I was in the hospital. A MRI of the brain, demonstrated MRA of the brain. The MRI showed a subacute stroke involving the left middle cerebral artery distribution. I had a minimal right facial asymmetry that improved considerably after the stroke. The neurological examination showed me symmetrical muscle power and tone. My deep tendon reflexes were symmetrical.

Humans, like other air-breathing vertebrates, have a double heart pumping action. With each heart contraction blood in the right ventricle is pumped through a pulmonary artery, leading to the lungs. As the blood passes through a vast capillary web in the lungs, carbon dioxide is released, and oxygen is acquired by the red cells. It is then returned to the left atrium and pumped by the left ventricle back into the systemic circulation.

In medical jargon: persistent areas of infarction in the left middle cerebral artery distribution with some persistent mass effect were not obviously increased. Why wait for illness before testing your doctor?

These painless, non-invasive technologies when you can gain access this technology. The members of National Stroke Association members of American Stroke Association's Stroke Initiative, a county wide program sponsored by local and regional hospitals, The American Heart Association and Advanced Screening for the education and prevention of stroke.

The "Y" is great, for me. They can give information with strokes, heart attacks, etc. They also allow me to encourage by a fee, as a disabled member. They know that I don't work, and want to make me healthy. They let me use their health fitness and equipment such as a track (around 22 equals one mile), treadmills, stationary bikes, weights, basketball gyms, aerobics rooms, swimming, etc. Locker rooms, showers, the whole health center.

Does the stroke make me a healthy, better writer? Or a better person? Maybe. I make it a point to invite to lunch, and to dinner for friends and professionals types. They are writers and photographers and former employers-employees. I don't ask them to plead a job! I'm still disabled, and I had health and dental insurance. But I want to what is out there. What is the business like, after I retired? I like to understand and hear friends working for money and jobs and whether they are happy... or not. Some are broke, some are well out. Some are retired, and disabled, and unemployed. Everyone tells me everything! They are employed, full time or part time, people moving, companies are hiring, companies are bankrupt, etc. It's interesting. I learn much in my friends and workers.

Are the stroke makes me a healthier and stronger? A little. I now have time to exercise, and to return to YMCA during work hours, at mostly around noon or early mornings. Twenty pounds has been deleted. Beer belly has been prohibited. One hundred forty pounds makes me better and healthier than 160 pounds at pre-stroke. I run five or six or seven miles twice a week during the winter, two or three miles at the "Y" carpeted track, and two or three miles on a treadmill. I bike 10 or 15 miles at a stationary bicycle. I was cherished for the Y during the wintertime. On the summer, I'll run three or five miles or 10 miles three or four times a week in the park or in the subdivision. If it's okay, warmer and sunny, it's no longer to go to the YMCA. On the bike path or streets I'll bicycle 10 miles or even 20 or 30 miles. I can pedal from my house to the beaches on the Lake St. Clair, one of the Great Lakes for Michigan. I take once daily for vitamins, it seemed that vitamin C is good for a stroke. Also a cup of coffee or orange juice, and then maybe yogurt (it gives calcium) and eat "other stuff". An anti-cholesterol for Cheerios for breakfast. In my home, I buy fruit to have a nutritious snack. Although cholesterol fears have caused American per capita egg consumption to drop from 400 to 250 per years, no research has ever shown that persons who eat more eggs have more heart attacks than people who eat fewer eggs, said one researcher. A healthy diet plan is worthless if people won't stick to it. Runner's World polled a group of ultramarathoners and Ironman triathletes to find out what they like to eat during their 8- to 24-hour races. They scored:

- Potatoes. Not french fried, but baked or boiled. An almost perfect for food in order to its carbohydrates.
- Chicken noodle soup. Not surprising. It's a very nutritious complex – and good for you.
- Rice cakes. High in carbs, fairly high in potassium. It tastes like nothing.
- Watermelon. Almost pure water, a good source of potassium and sugar.
- Bananas. The second for the list of fruits. They're good for potassium and sugar.

And no smoking. I was always against that. Both of my sisters smoke. It's a pack a day as most stroke survivals. A 60-year-old friend once said he smoked cigarettes at least a pack daily. Get rid of it. Simple, for me. But everyone: GET RID OF IT! They're #1 for all stroke survivors, all heart disease victims, and so on. A 50-year study published the first study firmly linking cigarette smoking to lung cancer and the most detailed and long-term results ever of the health effects of smoking. A life of smoking cigarettes will be, on average, 10 years shorter than a life without it. You knew that, right?

Another friend watched his mother and father get older, both of them smokers, breathing oxygen in tanks. The same thing killed from my neighbor and an uncle: emphysema, a chronic lung disease which oxygen and carbon dioxide are exchanged with the blood. Symptoms include short-windedness, very slow expiration of the breath, and whistling sounds during expiration. As the disease progresses, death may ultimately result of lung or heart failure. Already, you smoke cigarettes? Why?

Marriage is blissful, divorce is awful. I know. The sad case makes me sick. It was a marriage, 19 years, and she was gone – literally. She was a chapter in my life and my book. Marriage was sunny, warm and fun. She is gone, too. She was away from our life, her job, our house, our belongings, her boyfriend. I wrote this time at a meeting for aphasia:

"I have an occasional depression that makes a gloomy day.
I can't not think of my divorce and my wife. She is going now.
Dark and black. Is she coming back?"

It was terrible to not having my wife, capable of having a stroke and the virtual problems of communication and speech. I do think of the best of times. I once said, "I loved you." Now, I feel like you've gone even after I needed you here. Well, that's life. I don't really dwell. My son still lives with me, my daughter too, and I sleep in my home – I didn't care of my house. It was too big. I bought and moved in my condo. My wife does not understand aphasia. It's not her problem. Divorce it was harder. For a year it was still awful. After two years I had a good life, and the divorce was good, too. I went through the awful truth, acting at the courthouse with only my lawyer and my sister to hear from me for my sort of translator. I wrote my legal name in the divorce papers. I paid for my lawyer. I knew one word: divorce. I didn't know. I didn't care. I had a seminar on how to live without a marriage for eight weeks. It was ok. I needed eight months or eight years!

I don't cry myself for suffering my stroke. Stroke isn't a terrible cancer or a heart attack, I said. Some people have a stroke or aphasia from a year as long as all your life – and they are able to live anyway, with a life that is tough but possible. "Expect change, it's not always bad. Things may be different and different can be okay." I read this sentence construction in one day in therapy: "She's not coming back." It was the single, most important step in my therapy.

Chapter 5

Your support network

The three areas are your own reactions, your support network and your employees. My six months for 2003 has taken its stroke. Or that really means the word "aphasia." There was no calendar, no month, no year as it takes a date for me. Aphasia does not look for any calendar. It doesn't have a date. Today is not Monday, TGIF Friday is canceled, weekends or vacation were on the backburner. It's not a week, or two weeks before sore throats or stomach aches or broken bones can be better. Nothing is wrong with the throat. There is not a lozenge, not liquid medicines. You can't sing, like if it sounds an Irish brogue or an Italian opera or an American rock 'n roll. It won't work with the machinery, just won't receive any information. I wasn't lame, no bad left arm or right, not blocked vision, right leg or left leg with a brace that does not walk or run or skip ropes. It was just speaking, that's all. It really means for my career is an editor and publisher is finished. I was 100% disabled.

It was over it when checking out from the St. John Macomb Hospital. My therapists, conferences, meetings, and classes started at the clock hands finishing the stroke. My aphasia took my life. Hands gripped my throat, and the words were terrible. I had a dream with the sentences, giving them shorter and longer, reading pages as they're a puzzle. A number of several insights came to me: a job; a divorce; and stress along with all those things involving aphasia. Almost two years I'm still working, with attending conferences, meetings, classes, etc.

We have to self-serve our joined aphasics. Some can't speak. Some can't walk, or in wheelchairs. Some are brought the meetings with their caregivers. Some were in hospitals, having their strokes just two weeks ago, some years after it. The family will be told after they communicate with patients through the use of gestures. We'll say, "Tell your name. Tom. T-o-m. Say it. That's right. Your name is Tom." They are intelligent. They just can't speak. For a meeting, patients will provide with information to help them become effective partners in their recovery, and how to help protect against a future stroke. Have another stroke? That's scary! 42% of male stroke survivors have a second stroke within five years of the first. The stroke survivors have the right to the pursuit of happiness (the bill of rights) which includes:

- Free of labels (survivors or victors, not victims)
- Free of blame or guilt for having caused our disease
- Afforded the identity and dignity of first and foremost being a contributor to society
- Able to obtain as much information about stroke recovery
- Allowed to express our feelings with family and friends
- Able to establish a partnership with our physicians and others
- The necessary days after a stroke to discover what we can and cannot do in our former job

I am damaged. It's time if I said that. I won't get "normal" whatever that means. My job was gone. I was incapacitated.

In a conference for an American Stroke Association targets "our multiyear goal to reduce the risk of stroke by 25% before the year 2010." Well, that's one of my sights. I won't to be one of the 25% – as my term – composting. Growing like the daisies. Hippocrates called it the stroke, or plesso, for "thunderstruck." How do brain attacks and heart attacks differ? A couple of things: the sensitivity of a brain has a lack of oxygen; namely, as a heart attacking, which lasts many minutes. The reaction of a brain to injury has a rapid, "counter productive" chemical reactions, swelling in a closed space and the propensity for blooding. The heart is neither severe nor as rapid "counter productive." The time frames for the surviving a brain is three hours, with its heart as much as 12 hours. The propensity for blooding into the brain (10%) equals a heart propensity as less than 1% for bleeding into the brain. The asymptomatic carotid disease equals 1.3%, with the vascular death of 3.4%. Minor stroke is 6.1% is for the stroke, only 3.2% versus vascular death; 9% for major stroke, compared 3.5% for vascular death.

Someone, somewhere has written about their lifetime: "The stroke took my mobility and aphasia stole my nouns." My mobility is mine, and my nouns are mine too; but stroke can be the door up to aphasia. It lands upon my guest room. With a key to the lock. A noun is fairly simple. They give me cardboard cards like a sailboat, a clock, a dog like a golden retriever. I thought, "Well, that's easy. I'm not a dummy. But linking together, that's what the words that are empty. I can't get their handle, to put before and after, adverbs or adjectives or conjunctions. That's my problem." Notice, I thought it, but *never* saying it.

When a health practitioner asks you if your stroke has a problem with your right arm, or a left leg, or a blind eye. The brain becomes a single, gigantic problem. Some patient completely lost her taste after her stroke. She said it felt her teeth were decaying, and she strangled a lot. You had a stroke. A leg, an arm, an eye, a voice – they weren't communicating… that's the dilemma.

An application for a Special Petition for Appointment of Conservator stated: A physical illness or disability; the adult has property that will not be wasted or dissipated unless proper management is provided; the adult or his/her dependents are in need of money for support, care, and welfare and protection is necessary to obtain or provide money.

No adult keeps my money from being wasted, or "dissipated." No conservator never helps me with money for medical support, child care, etc. or rarely (if ever) managed my household, my lover, my car and my two teenagers. You can always be firm. Tell the judge it is time to get rid of the conservator. You can do it. Bark enough if you can speak before the judge. Or write it. Confidence and firm words are called in the courthouse. Barkin' dog!

It stated: The adult petitioner is mentally competent but due to age or physical informity (and) is unable to manage his/her property. It adds: "Patient recently had a stroke leading to right hemiparesis. The patient is aphasic, unable to communicate, he is disoriented and has poor memory. Judgement and insight, poor." Excuse me? Unable to communicate? I was disoriented? Not six weeks or six months after my stroke. Under my rights (why do I need my own rights?) it states you have the right to secure, at your own expense, an independent evaluation of your condition. If you cannot afford to pay for the evaluation, the court will approve reasonable costs to public expense. Under nature, purpose and legal effect of appointment of conservator. A guardian is a person who is appointed by a court to help an individual to make personal decisions when the individual is unable to make such decisions. If a guardian is appointed for you, the guardian would make decisions for you that you now may make for yourself. For example, the guardian could decide such things as what *medical care you receive and where you live.*

I looked at "guardian" under the dictionary. It said: a superior of a Franciscan monastery. So odd! I will have a guardian who is the superior from a Franciscan monastery who does my expenses! And as far as "where you live"... barkin' dog! No guardian or conservator is going to say where I am living. I was, and then, checked a report as a mental incompetent. This was in July 9, 2002, a few days from my stroke. You have the right to a trial by jury. Sound like a police-drama, Dragnet? You have the right to request that the hearing be closed to the public. You have the right to present evidence at the hearing.

A report by the National Ethics Committee of the Veterans Health Administration (VHA) provides clinicians with practical information about decision-making capacity and how it is assessed. Number 1: Decision-making capacity and legal competency are the same. Number 2: Lack of decision-making capacity can be presumed when patients go against medical advice. Patients with certain psychiatric disorders lack decision-making capacity. A stroke patient it's a commonplace. They don't have disorders and don't lack decision-making capacity. Only mental health experts can assess decision-making capacity.

A letter written by Lionel Glass M.D., The Neurology Clinic, in August 9, 2002, "He developed the acute onset of, what appeared to have been, a left middle cerebral artery distribution stroke... His speech has evidence of a rather significant expressive aphasia." However, he states, "It is my impression that Mr. Bas should do well with extensive, intensive speech therapy."

My family physician Dr. Donald Cucchi wrote: "Mr. Bas... operates a vehicle, handles our finances and maintains own home. He is oriented to time, space and surroundings." I even voted Mr. Bush. "His answers are appropriate to questions and this office feels that he may terminate his conservatorship, if the court so agrees." Set up a chalk up for Dr. Cucchi! I've talked to many stroke survivors – stroke victors – have a stroke 10, 15, 20 years, and more: Janis, Philip, Bill, Dave, Mary, Paul, Edward, Mike, Paul, and Glen. I wrote their words. Here's what I learned.

Janis, Bill, Dave, Phil, and ...

Janis was founded the aphasia group, as different from the stroke survivors. She who is a spark plug with plenty of activity. She wonderfully orchestrated the aphasia group, keeping laughs and the stream of a roomful of meetings. She will proudly that she was identified "Paula" in "Pathways," the book by Susan Adair Ewing and Beth Pfalgraf. It was only, the book tells us, after Paula's first memories after two craniotomy surgeries. It had arteriovenous malformation (AVM) which had her with difficulty as speech and movement. This was 1979, more than 20 years ago, over three years she was in a great deal of pain, and she was having many seizures. After much despair, Paula (Janis) was transferred to another hospital to begin rehabilitation. She was a patient in a rehabilitation unit. She said, the rehabilitation unit was terrible and she was depressed. In 1981, she was in the hospital for four months. A doctor told those that she wasn't communicating, that she probably not even understand you. Fortunately, her family helped her and stood by her. She has been "cured" since she was discharged four months in December of 1982 (more than 20 years). She has been as slaying the aphasic dragon since her recovered life. She is an artist, who paints with watercolors and pottery at the age of 54. "The future promised far greater challenges and opportunities," wrote the book, written in 1990. She promised great challenges, 15-20-25 years from then!

Philip, of St. Clair Shores, gave an encouraging to me for my first meeting. Always nattily dressed in a turtleneck or a sweater and a sportscoat, his beard looking somewhat a college professor, he has a cane and a brace, and he came up with the meeting's name: New Beginnings. He has aphasia, apraxia, dysarthria (speech impairment characterized slurring lips, teeth and breathing from a muscular weakness), anomia (word recall impairment), and dysphagia (swallowing impairment).

Phil and Jan were engaged at one time. "We're going to elope, I think," joked Phil The almost-married couple had an unhappy one. It's not easy for aphasic survivors. They were not married. Janis is one of our veterans. She said she got butterflies for her nervous stomach. It was another lost hint. It's bad with two aphasics, told Phil to me. It was hard to communicate with each other. They are still serious about their aphasia meetings and helping others who suffer from their strokes and aphasia, and seeking their support. "It's so hard, but you can get better," Jan stated. I am so sorry for them, and I truly hope their lives were kind and good.

Paul, a stroke victor, is much a speaker today. He reads "Simplified Sentence Skills," one for writers and not just patients with aphasia. He wanted to know what they were taught and what directed them. Paul was an electrical technician before working at General Motors Coach & Truck, then he worked as a computer technician. He worked for Control Data for 17 years, and for 15 years as EDS. As wife, Judy, works as a private rehabilitation business. From all his seven uncles died from heart fatalities, and his father suffered heart killing him at 1967. He had his stroke in 1996. Doctors said he would not get any better. Everyone has a doctor proscribed a ruin fate and a foreboding doom to his/her stroke. His language today is almost perfect. He spent a lot of time practicing his talk to his dogs: five St. Bernard and one German Shepherd and three cats, but people don't talk to the cats. They're apathetic (cats are thought to understand just as many words, they just choose not to acknowledge them.)

Dave admits he does not have aphasia. He is disabled from a stroke with a dissipated vision. He is unable to drive. He told me, at 47, he had a recent divorce also. He went to a few aphasia meetings, and he said, "You're heroes, everyone else. I understand what you live after a stroke." He is a physical therapist for a volunteer at St. Joseph Hospital. "I have a good image of what you have," he said. "You can really be proud, with a dilemma for strokes." He lives in a condominium close to the hospital. He didn't drive a car. Dave had a stroke, he does not have aphasia. He feels that he is not failed or futile at all. Dave was partially blind (the eyes are fine, he reassures, they just getting the information in his brain) he is confident, assured. You have to ignore objects on that blinded side. He had a problem reading, dressing, even walking. You accidentally move into furniture and a closed door, if you won't see it. You won't neglect your weaker side. Blind is not new to a stroke survivor.

Mike, 54, is a journalist and keeps The Aphasia Club with a newsletter on his Dell computer. He had a "sick leave" from his job. He was a writer at one and a half years for public relations at Chrysler Corp. Before, he was a WKAR public radio reporter, a Flint Journal newspaper, the Associated Press, and Detroit News as an editor. He had an emergency heart surgery in November 1997 and 10 days later he suffered a massive stroke, both incidents being caused by unexplained blood clots. "I am better than I began the stroke five years ago." He jokes, "Now, in 20 or 30 years, I'll be complete better." He has "retired" from skin diving, although he and his wife, Sue, spent a vacation around the Caribbean (Grand Turk in the Bahamas, Jamaica, Grand Cayman, Belize and off the Venezuela Bonaire). Mike has 3-4 printed pages a thumbnail, with other survivors written their lives after strokes and/or aphasia. My profile was written in July 2004. "Since his stroke, he had written a book on aphasia, and he runs and plays tennis in his spare time. Noting what he learned from the conference, he said exercise and maintaining a healthy weight are important for living after having a stroke." I was "famous" in my article after 15 minutes.

Mike still likes swimming and scuba diving, reads a lot and (almost) never misses an aphasia meeting, two or three in a week. Mike and Sue went to the National Aphasia Association convention in Florida, and later, national conventions to Ypsilanti, Mich. and Washington D.C. Five years a loo-oong time, I thought. I don't like to acquaint aphasia with another 20 or 30 years! There was a motivational speaker, Lynn Serper. She was an author with the book "Brainstorming: the Serper Method of Brain Recovery, Recovery and Vitality," and she has her own web site, www.brainvitality.com. "Each time you hear normal language," she said, "your ears will teach your language system how to speak. Remember, every conversation MUST have a listener!"

Mary was my friend and she was at my many meetings. She had her stroke after a terrible accident driving her car some 15 years ago. Today she is 40-plus, and she has a wheelchair. She had a closed head injury in addition to breaking her neck, crushed heel, collapsed lung, traechotomy, knee surgery, a halo inserted onto her neck fusion, Groshong catheter, feeding tube, several operations and surgeries, etc. "At the time of my accident in '89, I was one in 1,000 to survive the accident. I had barely survived," she said. "I thank God every day for giving me the determination and courage and strength to endure many painful tests and operations and be able to live such a fulfilling, fun, independent, joyful life. I got divorced shortly after I came home from my accident so it's been a little more than 15 years for me. I had a couple relationships since that but nothing that lasted more than a year and it's been a long time so I've become very independent and close to God who is my peace and comfort and refuge." She can cook, exercises and keeps busy at her own home, which she has at it for eight years. She supervises her house, repairs and additions, and she single-handedly landscaping and gardening an acre in the backyard.

She keeps her house clean by washing the floor on her knees. She sings at a choir for Christ United Methodist Church in Fraser, Michigan. She has divorced from 13 years. She is at the aphasia and stroke meetings, volunteers at the children's hospital and senior citizen housing. She gardens at a "big yard" even in the middle of the also big city. She cultivates lots of flowers: crocuses, tulips, lilies, black eyed susan, phlox, lupine, dianthus, zinnia, peonies, petunia, marigold, hollyhock, mums, impatiens, aster, clematis, yucca, trumpet vine, morning glories, salvia, hibiscus, roses, daisies, red hot pokers, coreopsis, cosmos, wildflowers, calendula, lilac weigela, gladiola, liatris, dahlia, coral bells, begonia, geranium, astilbe, hosta, canna, asuria, jasmine, dames rocket, sweet william, verbena, pansies, blood grass, zebra grass, mandivilla, sweet pea, ranunculus, ice plant, daffodil, tithonia, iris. She has trees, too... cherry, apple, pear, peach, plum, willow, forsythia, redbud. If you want, she can grow your own plants from seeds! Her garden has a window for the sunlight during winter, and is quite thriving and comfortable. She gives a fertilizer, called "Miracle-Gro." Mary gives us a poem, which she reads, as the result of a once waitress. Her poem "Stiffed" on wages and tips, mused the waitress.

I went to the table to pick up my tip
I lifted the napkins and stuck out my lip
I gave the best service that I knew how
I watched as he gorged himself like a cow
I gave him more water, more butter, more tea
I was everything that a waitress could be
I was pleasant, I smiled and fulfilled every need
As to why there's no tip... I haven't a lead

Everyone is sure that only older people have strokes. Just not true. In 1999, 35-year-old Kevin Gardner, according from the American Heart Association, just completed a 15-mile bike ride when he got a severe headache. Six hours later he had a blurred vision and slurred speech. He knew that he had warning strokes. A million stroke survivors have suffered little or no long-lasting disability from their strokes. Another two million live with the crippling and lifelong disabilities of paralysis, loss of speech, and poor memory.

Lisa, 30 years-plus, was in Clinton Township, Mich., close to my aphasia and stroke meetings. She had her stroke more than a year ago. A poet also, Lisa wrote, "The Angel's Voice." "Your Friendship begins to mean all the more, if Fear and Worry might have caused sleep to be short, or when the day of the heart has been to long," it began.

Many of our aphasics write songs, poems, short stories, and books. They are trying to hear their lost words. It's easier writing down their feelings and it's harder to talk to their friends and their relatives. Everybody has a story to tell. Aphasics are encouraged to write them down. Start by writing a diary or a daily journal. Take a class or have a writing convention or conference. Have your work with copies and give it to your meetings. If you read your work, it's easier than talking on the cuff, or better than giving a speech with your friends or acquaintances. I'm scared even with my friends – a two minute speech would be a jumbled link of words, rather than sentences. "Blogs" have become one of their fastest growing segments of the Internet. A blog ("web log") can create an online journal for publishing. Enough of your thoughts, suffering and opinions can be seen with other readers. Enjoy them!

Glen has a big laugh, and a career as a lawyer. He brings a scrapbook and a school yearbook for the meetings. The scrapbook has his wife, a Vietnamese, which he sought in the trip for the USO. His photos saw the wife, his family, the many bicycles in the street, and the houses and buildings. He was always carrying his digital camera for aphasia meetings.

Bill always gives us a chuckle; he reminds a joke written a lot to us which he resolves. The jokes are sometimes from Reader's Digest. It takes a lot of reciting, remembering, maybe five minutes for a joke. You can "hear" his smiles, his pronouncing and selecting every single word, every sentence. From inner smiles and outer smiles, too, you hear from his best jokes. He and his wife, with Mike and Sue (and the author of this book), were in Tampa, Fla. at the fourth convention of the National Aphasia Association, cosponsored the University of South Florida.

At another stroke meeting, one at St. John North Shores Hospital, Dick is the one to first to laugh and giving a joke and saying, "Hello, how are you doing?" If you had three weeks or so unable to see a meeting, he wants to know what happened. Where have you been? You're ok? he asked. At one of the meetings, he talks and talks. Our therapist says, "He once didn't speak a word, at the meetings. But suddenly it just came out. When it suddenly started, he's never missed out!" We were playing a word game, then we will give a hint, either a word or a phrase. "Yacht." We will say, "It's a big boat, or a ship. Like very expensive." Dick is the one for a word: "Cruise ship, yacht." He guessed until the word has been out.

There is always a favorite name game, with clues for familiar actors and actresses: Marilyn Monroe, for example. Their movies, they were born, dead, etc. Sometimes a name is hard to remember, although they can name the tip of the tongue. "Fred Astaire" was the common actor's name. He was a dancer. He was an old timer from the black and white movies. But what was his name? "He was... he was... he was... they thought... that, that... " The stuttering and the name would not come out. I told them, "His name is the same as the Flintstones." The name is Fred, is that a clue? Still nothing. Second name, walking with fingers gestured from the first floor up to the second floor: "The stairs." They couldn't know it, or if they knew it they wouldn't work lips or throat; or the brain wouldn't make the connection. Shout, yell, clap your hands, bark, howl... even talk. Say it, "Fred Astaire."

Another person, Marge, is a regular contributor to our meetings at St Joseph Hospital, north a few miles from St. John Hospital. She was a vocational nun. She is an artist and poet. She had a stroke and meets with her friends at the stroke support group once a month at St. Joseph Hospital. "In the future, neurologists may prescribe friendship and a housekeeper," a newsletter said. "... the number of friends stroke patients have and whether they receive and in-home help are the best indicators for predicting another stroke."

Ronald Johnson, black, 50ish, enjoys playing at casinos, but enjoys it when he makes money. Everyone is a gambler with disease or heart attack or stroke. When a younger woman was pretending that she was drinking milk, another word guessing game, Ronald guessed she was sipping wine. I said, "Ronald, you like to gamble at the casinos and drink wine!" They laughed. Sarah is a young student, 20-plus, in a speech therapy program at Wayne State University, and Adam and Rochelle. Marcy, a student, just got married with her boyfriend in Las Vegas. Chad McCarney, MA, CCC-SLP, joins the students and his students too. Chad has tried to meet with a social worker finding a job from an aphasia patient. They were my friends. Julie Klocke and Cheryl Pietraszewski, are speech-language pathologists (therapists), at St. Joe and St. John hospitals, respectively, and always makes us sure that we have something for eating at meetings – pizzas, cake, cookies for Valentine's Day, and for Mother's Day. As Klocke says, "A scrumptious good time." They're all busy at feeding us. There are plenty of social and entertainment meetings-conferences. The Stroke Connection Retreat is in weekends in July "a getaway weekend for stroke survivors, caregivers and family members of all ages" at Camp Cavell, a YWCA camp on the sandy-rocky shores of Lake Huron in Lexington, Michigan. A "Spring Fling" is an annual gathering of southeastern Michigan stroke clubs, including contributions from members and clubs, music and entertainment, as "well as encouraging talks, prizes and lunch." Another meeting, Cane and Able (it's about capability, not disability) holds its 21st anniversary dinner. It was your opportunity to speak your mind, share with the group, talk to them, encourage or remember friends, or just say, 'Thanks, I'm happy to still be here.'" Cane and Able had a speaker for its twice monthly meetings, sometimes a field trip to see a member's house or a game with the Detroit Tigers or at an art gallery.

At a Warren, Mich. there was a stroke meeting on Wednesdays every week, 10 a.m. till noon. It's only four miles from me, four miles from the St. John Hospital. Its name is "Change of Pace Stroke Club." They provide social and recreational activities, is a part of the city's Parks & Recreation department. Call the departments of your cities, hospitals, speech and language departments at the university, etc. You can name it, trips, discussions, dinners, parties, exercise, shopping, billiards, playing cards with euchre and pinochle. Their motto: A means of promoting knowledge about stroke, its causes and effects and how to prevent stroke. Their newsletter keeps a calendar and a column with "under the weather" sending "cards of encouragement to our friends who are not able to join us." A stroke club is a group of people with common concerns, they come together to offer support and mutual encouragement. It's a way of socializing and learning from others, friends Roy and Ernie and Clifford. There is a meeting probably near your home, whenever and where ever. I have *lots* of friends!

Said someone in an obituary, "There was music before Ray Charles and there's music after Ray Charles." I thought about it. There was a life before stroke and after stroke.

They are all my acquaintances or friends, dozens of them, with strokes or aphasia. "Finally, the use of supportive stroke groups or clubs can be of great value in maintaining levels of speech performance and especially morale," read *Working With Apraxic Clients*.

"The treatment strategies of aphasia are inevitably different from those for apraxia and dysarthria, even though the broader management issues may overlap," Working With Apraxic Clients, by Susan Huskins, who worked in apraxia patients. "Aphasia is a disorder of language, hence the rationale of treatment is aimed at improving language performance in all modalities – auditory, lexic, oral, and graphic (heard, read, spoken, and written language)." Motor exercises in the context of appropriate language therapy. Apraxic clients are also aphasic to a degree. Apraxia of the paralyzed or left hand has been reported many times in clients who have a right aphasia. Features apply:

1) Syntactic errors present
2) Morphological errors present
3) Semantic errors present

4) Word-finding errors present
5) Phonological (the science of speech sounds) errors present (the selection and sequencing errors occur)
6) Persevere occurs at the level of words
7) Persevere occurs at sound level
8) Phonological errors reflected in writing
9) Linguistic errors reflected in all modalities (linguistics is the study of speech including units, nature, structure and modification)
10) Auditory comprehension, discrimination and monitoring impaired

In addition, apraxic including the groping for articulatory postures, a groping, frequent repeats and attempts at self-correction, speech generally labored and slower, the production of non-English sounds and sequences, etc.

At one point, "but spontaneous recovery often results in dramatic improvement... however, after the first month, the client is still equally impaired, the outlook is obviously poor. A period of diagnostic therapy may be necessary to discover if the client has any potential for recovery of speech or language, or for learning an alternative method of communication." Editors could be a problem unless an *alternative method of communication* is appeared. An alternative? Maybe, sign language? Telecommunications, or telepathy? Communication with smoking, fires and blankets, like the Indians did?   At one aphasic meeting, the word was given at three survivors. The word was *angry*. They were angry, they said, for not talking. They are angry because they don't have the insight to lend a word, or a sentence. The frustration of aphasia may cause irritability. I am feeling angry with the chapter in the book, for my divorce workshop or seminar. For aphasics, they are angry because (I honestly got these examples from my acquaintances):

Are you talking because of your stroke, or are you going to get better?

You had a stroke just six months ago? Should you be playing volleyball? ("No, you better phone an ambulance, RIGHT NOW!")

How are you doing? (I'm actually dying. And how are you?) Neurons are dead in your brain. Let's hope your brain gets better. (Me, too.)

You had a stroke? Was it a bad one, or just "slightly" or "medium" for a stroke?

It seemed to me that I am still alive and living after my stroke. That's the hardest thing. Stroke finished the end, but aphasia was not an ending – it's just getting ready. I find a way of thinking, a means of writing and reading. Reading a book can be difficult with too many pages, especially if it doesn't have any of my material or information. I'm reading slowly, two pages, sometimes three pages, and I shelve the book if it's not a good one. Prior-stroke, I read 30-40 pages in one sitting. The writing was hard, too. Sometimes I finish reading a book or a magazine piece at first the last page. Then I re-read it, the middle and first pages in the beginning. This is a no-no, told the author! Written by journalists, from each and every instructor taught it, leading an article or a story. Hook them. Because the readers only read the first sentence, or the first paragraph. A lead is from a journalistic phrase. Get them interested. Make them curious.

But I wrote my book, one that was written before I had my stroke, on the subject of indoor air quality. The rewrite, which was not hard, was almost easier. It was a chapter on mold, and the publisher wanted a new version. The book was titled Indoor Air Quality; A Guide for Facility Managers. I wrote my book with all the information from magazine articles and reports or interviews. The subject, mold, was done a long time ago in heating-ventilation-air conditioning trade magazines. An old subject but new information with my readers. But aphasia has been difficult to me, for a lot of reasons. In the book, indoor air quality, it was easier. I deleted it or added it for new information or data. But my truly original book, "Barkin' Dog; How to Talk with Aphasia," was to be written, and rewritten, editing and re-editing. Twice or three times or four times. Not all sentences were unclearly. I had to rewrite again and again. I didn't know what to write. One year after a stroke, I couldn't pronounce the words

"Sterling Heights" and "August," as well as the word "aphasia." I wrote "the long, bad road" was simple enough, but I didn't have the words, sentences, and paragraphs to make sense.

People said once my writing was simple and straightforward with my books and articles. I wrote to my readers as they were reading about their favorite subject. "While action on indoor air quality (IAQ) has increased dramatically in recent years, the roots of IAQ awareness go back to ancient times." It was simple enough. My writing career was 25 years plus. I wrote hundreds (thousands?) of articles and stories. The wording was familiar. I wrote it but I can't re-read them, in advance from six months my stroke. Since the stroke, I wrote my book the first time and then I wrote it the second way a little better, and a third time and fourth time. The problems and syntax were worst from the first version. They stunk!

I felt like I could contribute to an aphasia book. Those attended a stroke conference many were the health community. But very few were editors, and fewer had stroke survivors. How can communicate with your doctor? Can he or she write a book? I can write, and see what no one has seen. A seminar on "How to Get Published" at a local university, instructors taught professional presentations to develop publishable manuscripts. The seminar attends to writers on how to style, format and appearance. Format and appearance contributes to the pleasure or pain of the reader or reviewer. And, lastly, writing is sometimes poor, and the material poorly organized. I write what I really enjoy: my life, my friends, my writing career. I want to know, learn, and read about it, and have convictions about my message.

Chapter 6

Write, write, write

Write, write, write. That's what Lynn Lazarus Serper, Ed.D., in her "Everyday Survival – Brainstorming," believed. "Keep a daily journal about anything – your life, someone else's life, something you read, an event you experienced, news of the day – *anything*. Write or copy one word or a page of words by hand or on a computer." She suggests work on it for 30 minutes in the morning and 30 minutes later that day. One hour. I will keep writing every two hours in the morning, after I walked the dog Sammy, grocery shopping, eating lunch, etc., and two hours in the afternoon – sometimes an hour for evening. "You *will* see progress!" she remarked. I really and truly pray with seeing progress. My first speech classes at Wayne State University were beginning with my second education. "The Speech and Language Center has two primary purposes. The purposes are to provide speech therapy services to you and to provide clinical training for our students who are seniors or graduate students majoring in speech-language pathology. Time is spent daily, not only by your clinician, but also by the faculty of the university, preparing for each session. We do this is to ensure the finest clinical services to you." Help me! I thought. Give me my voice. Don't see me a picture of a sailboat, a house, a car, or an alarm clock! That's simple. I know what they are!

I saw a book, "Coping with Aphasia." I have a problem with this book. *Coping With Aging, a Series* was written to an audience for senior citizens. Our meetings, often, are in the senior citizens' buildings. That's nice, but... a lot of our aphasics are younger, maybe 35 or 45 years old. Older people do not generally have only aphasia – only people with aphasia had strokes. Older patients have Alzheimer's disease and dementia, but why senior citizens have aphasia? Why have a book or tapes on older people with "Tooth and Your Aging Dental" with the Coping With Aging Series. "The books in the Coping With Aging Series are written for men and women coping with the challenges of aging and disease, and for their families and other caregivers." I think it's a mistake: disease and aging have little to do with aphasia. If you're older, you have strokes or heart attacks or disease. That does not compute. "Caregivers" are offering their patients with a life without speaking or reading. Maybe this is a book written for speech pathologists, or caregivers. "Striving to improve!" it tells the readers. A patient could be addressed to my assumption, not just written to caregivers. Tell them (the stroke victors) what is coming, and what is progressing. "The Secret Life of the Brain," written by Richard Restak, MD deals with the brain. As the baby's brain, children with a growing mature brain, throughout as the adult and aging brain. It's probably good, as it goes. But the stroke is on page 181, right in the end of the book. Under the chapter of the book is "Second Flowering; The Aging Brain." Aging? Second flowering? It seems odd, to having a new brain as the baby, versus the aging, stroke-prone, unhealthy brain. As though it's unhealthy, along with cancer and heart disease. Do neurons have senility? It's easier in chapters, a week program developed a PBS-awarded series. But it's incorrect, for the brain. Stroke comes in brains as young as 20s, 30s or 40s. It is not "the aging brain." Brains are replenished and renovated. The memory, Alzheimer's and dementia (called senility another senior citizen's enigma) are not classified as the stroke. That second flowering reminds me of that term *composting,* or the final of a "third flowering" –as in "dirt." MRI revealed a survivor with her an infarction of the right thalamus. The damage of her right thalamus reacted to her somatosensory cortex in the right parietal lobe. It caused a loss of all sensation to her left face, arm, leg, and trunk. Her vision was lost of her left side. It's not Alzheimer's disease or dementia. She was not aging. She was 43 years old.

My speech pathologist mused my neurons as they "are now dead." My neurons are DEAD. They must be replaced, or grown (perhaps we help them with composting). I will call that the neurons are "sleepy." They needed something more like an alarm clock, or jumper cables coupled with a "Diehard" 12-volt battery. If they are dead, they are... well, *dead*. They are expired, deceased, departed. The hippocampus in the stem cells contribute neurons. It cements the response to the threat into long-term memory. No one can say which neurons can do it, or what they can move. (Helpful hints: The only thing is that a hippocampus in the brain is different from a hippopotamus in the swamp. It's funny because they're similar! Actually, they are close to the Greek language. Hippocampus means seahorses, and a "sea horse" whose shape they resemble.) A new understanding of fear has also led to pharmacological treatments for post-traumatic stress disorder. Autonomic reaction have beat-blockers keep memory from forming deeper grooves in the brain, making post-traumatic stress symptoms (like a stroke) less severe. The ultimate goal is to find a way of performing virtual experiments than can quickly a discovery of new medical treatments and reducing their cost. A few of these pharmaceutical companies have already offering such services, but the accuracy of their models has not been verified by scientific peer review. The goal is not perfect but reliable approximation. Engineers can design an airplane in a computer but virtually without ever building one. The researchers can't explain how air will flow in a realistic way. The Alliance for Cellular Signaling regulates in the models of immune systems, such as E. coli and influenza. The pioneers will be a genetic programming for a stroke or a heart attack. A scientist like Pasteur will be a computer-brain technician (different from a neurologist) or gene engineer.

One of the great clinical writers

A doctor who is "one of the great clinical writers of the 20th century" was the speaker at a spring conference on aphasia. Oliver Sacks, wrote "The Man Who Mistook His Wife for a Hat." He also wrote *The Awakening*, a book turned to a movie (the title is *The Awakenings*, a plural was inserted), starring Robin Williams and Robert DeNiro. The patients for the neurologist (Williams) given them a sort of jumper cables for giving him dopamine (or seronin and norepinephrie which are neurotransmitters.) for a drug therapy. Dr. Oliver Sacks wrote the remarkable account of a group like Rip van Winkles, survivors of the great sleeping sickness epidemic which struck just after first World War. The patients before had a long, long sleep. They were unresponsive. They were deemed unconscious and given up as hopeless until these patients were prescribed the drug L-DOPA. The patients had an explosive, "awakening" effect that brings back an absence of nearly 40 years. Dr. Sacks tells the moving story of this extraordinary individual, courageous and tragic, with questions of health, suffering, and the human condition.

A second, smaller, self-contained battery for an automobile industry, marketers announced the battery can "wake up" a dead (or sleeping) car or truck. What if the battery goes dead in your car or truck, or in the middle of the night? What you do then? What do you do from the same as a heart attack, having a sudden stroke? Sacks' biography, was titled "Uncle Tungsten." No, Uncle Tungsten has nothing to do with aphasia. But it's good nevertheless in a sort of scientific or medical best-sellers. "I was not allowed to touch them once they were lit – they were sacred, I was told, their flames were holy, not to be fiddled with. I was mesmerized by the little cone of blue flame at the candle's center – why was it blue? Our house had coal fires, and I would often gaze into the heart of a fire, watching it go from a dim red glow to orange, to yellow, and then I would blow on it with the bellows until it glowed almost white-hot. If it got hot enough, I wondered, would it blaze blue, be blue-hot? Did the sun and stars burn the same way? Why did they never go out? What were they made of?" Uncle Tungsten is truly renaissance for us, the scientific biography was his life. In from a back issue from Scientific American, Science News and Popular Science, there is reading on the numerous subjects from nuclear rockets to Milky Way galaxies – mechanical to engineering, medicine to chemistry to physics. Astronomy to aphasia, it becomes a black hole, a voodoo subject for me. So much information, so exciting! Stars, dark planets, nebulae – who can resist such a subject? Sacks, a neurosurgeon, wrote Uncle Tungsten just like his Uncle Dave. Sacks wrote his Uncle as "loved the density of the tungsten he made, and its refractoriness, its great chemical stability... This sense of extended family was one I knew and enjoyed as far back as memory goes... All of us, I could not help imagining, had a bit of the old man in us."

A right hemisphere, a left hemisphere and a cerebellum create the three sites of a stroke. The left "right" hemisphere carries a right-side paralysis, loss of vision in the right eye and, for me, problems in speaking and/or understanding the communications of others. Speech pathologists can speak a noun, that's easy, but two or threes nouns, add adjectives or a verb or pronouns, and a conjunction. They lost me. Depression and slowness, impaired thinking and temporary confusion can be equally distributed.

The right hemisphere can be emotional instability, dulled responsiveness, poor judgment, confusion, disoriented time and location, life-sided weakness or paralysis, etc. The cerebellum can be a loss of balance, dizziness or nausea and vomiting. I'll take the left hemisphere. Silent and quiet... a barkless dog! President Ford was hospitalized during a week in 2000. He suffered a brain-stem stroke at in most cases can be devastating or even fatal. He had a stroke in his late 60s, but survived age 89, a stroke victor. He bounced back with some minor balance problems.

Leonard LaPointe's "Adapting to Life with Aphasia" is a keynote speaker at the National Aphasia Association in Tampa in 2004. He is a professor in Communications Sciences and Disorders at Florida State University. Economic and financial times changed, LaPointe said. He described a "Titanic", a sudden and catastrophic shipwreck for stroke patients. Aphasia is after the iceberg. Aphasia altered relationships, employment and opportunity for stroke survivors. Many people are retired or disabled with after their stroke. Many are truly impoverished or retired before 60 years or even 50.

Research for coping strategies is meager, LaPointe said. There are plenty of reasons that need stroke survivors: emotional-personality effects; altered employment; altered leisure activity; change in living environment; altered relationships, etc. Some crucial questions need some patients in coping, quality of life, self-esteem, body image and identity. "When am I going to be me, or normal, again?" LaPointe said. "Never. It's a downsized life. Do you know that people having lunch at Taco Bell seems they know about tacos to understand about stroke or aphasia?" The illness "experience" is coping with chronicity – themes largely missing from the rehabilitation literature. Realization or denial, mourning or adaptation: that's what the patient feels. Shock or frozen feelings, or guilt and panic are used to leave a hospital after a stroke, with hostility or hating the life after – maybe months or years ago – the survivor's acceptance for compliance or "life is ok!"

A noun is a noun

Why is a noun just a noun? Any member of a class of words with combined with determiners. A clock is a clock. A picture of a sailboat, is a picture of just a sailboat. Four minus two equals two. A flash card: 18 divided by 6 equals 3. I know that. A dog is not a clock. But taking a noun is I will see a noun, maybe pictured a dog versus a clock versus a car. Two or three nouns will be just that. But linking them... that's the harder part. Broca's aphasia is thus characterized as a nonfluent aphasia. Affected people often omit small words like "is" "but" and "the." For example, the "Walk dog" means "I will take my dog for a walk." The same two words could mean, "The dog walked out of my backyard." Same difference. The fluent aphasia from Wernicke's they might add a word that means nothing. For instance, "The dog frimmed the bedroom." Frimmed? What do you mean? The dog walked? And I said "the bedroom"... do you mean the backyard? Or do you really mean the bedroom, versus the backyard? Words can be changed or altered for them to where or why or how to use them. Smaller words of speech may be omitted, making the message sound like a telegram. Words may be put in the wrong order. Dog eats food. Food eats dog! Grammar may be used incorrectly. I like my words. They're different or similar. It takes me a minute, two minutes or five minutes if you have time.

The convention for aphasia was different for me. I was in a stranger in a strange land. I was in a health or medical convention. Their names were r.n., ph.d, ma ccc. I didn't know the abbreviations. I never had the idea or never guessed what was the dictionary done as, like the dictionary said, impairment of the power to comprehend words: aphasia.

A report in a trade journal called for hurrying stroke patients to the hospital. But it seemed like a good idea. Quicker was better. "Getting to the hospital as soon as possible after a stroke," it read, "starts is key to warding off the potentially disabling effects," it wrote by Jennifer Warner and Michael Smith, MD. Because a survey showed that although people may know more about stroke warning signs than in the past, most people don't understand what actually increases the risk of having a stroke. Warning signs of a stroke are ironic: sudden numbness or weakness of the face, arm or leg, especially on one side of the body. My stroke was suddenly, instant to me. I was in the hospital three days with another week; the rehabilitation was two years and counting. Less than 90 minutes is critical with stroke. Some communities are improving the transporting, diagnosing or treating the stroke patients, but many don't have the staff or equipment to quickly treat stroke. Only 5% of stroke patients arrive at a hospital in time are to be treated with a clot-busting drug that can help reduce permanent brain damage and long term disability if given within three hours of the start of symptoms. Stroke is our #3 killer and a leading cause of series, long-term disability. But only 1% of Americans worry about it. Many think that living with a major stroke disability – such as being unable to talk or move one side of the body – would be worse than dying, but most don't think about stroke until it affects their family. We must implement stroke treatment protocols in every community or we'll see more stroke deaths or disability, and medical costs of stroke, nearly $50 billion per year will keep rising.

You can't hold your life before your stroke. Your life will be damaged or impaired. Expect a harder life. You won't have your career, you won't eat the things you want to, you won't get your close friends, maybe you won't exercise a lot or play the piano or play your bowling or golfing league. You can't expect to it ever be all right. Why not? Why can't I exercise and have a job? I refuse to have a different life. I can't have my life, but I refuse to have yet another life. My hobbies are still there. Think about it. Tell your therapists and your doctors you will have the same life.

My friends and I were always kidding about how we were smart. Another one, we laughed and called him, "The super (soooo-per) genius" like Wile E. Coyote in the Roadrunner cartoons. We told about each other, "Einstein." We were into general science, computers, astronomy, cars, books, magazines, travel, bikes and running, etc. We weren't senile, I hope. I was too young for dementia or Alzheimer's. For a stroke, it's different. I was not too young for having a stroke. My brain can't get on track. My communication headquarters is vacant. The hq has moved.

Drugs known as clot-busters have the potential to save the lives of untold people brought to emergency rooms after suffering strokes. But many doctors continue to use the drugs incorrectly, often with serious consequences. A report of 16 hospitals in Connecticut found that mistakes were made in the way the drugs were given to 97% of the stroke patients. The research found the records of 63 patients given thrombolytic (clot-busting) from 1996-98. They found a history of mistakes occurring throughout treatment, including screening at the time of admission, laboratory tests and interpretation of brain imaging. Patients were given the wrong dosages, or given the drugs too late, or were given the drugs even though they had a stroke that could be seriously worsened by giving clot-busters. They are drugs for ischemic strokes vs. a blood clot, not a hemorrhagic stroke. While not usually fatal, ischemic is a blockage of a blood vessel in the brain or neck. The most frequent cause of stroke and is responsible for about 80% of strokes. These blockages have three conditions, mainly the formation of a clot (thrombosis), the movement of the slot within a blood vessel in the brain or neck (embolism), or a severe narrowing called stenosis.

For the study, researchers surveyed about 2,000 residents of the greater Cincinnati area in 2000 and asked them to name at least three major warning signs for stroke. Then the researchers compared their results to a similar survey conducted in 1995.

In 2000, 70% of the respondents were able to correctly name at least one established warning sign of stroke, compared with only 57% in 1995. But when it came to correctly naming at least one major risk factor, there was only a 4% increase in awareness from 1995 to 2000 (68% to 72%).

The results appeared in the January 15, 2003 issue of The Journal of the American Medical Association. Study researcher Alexander T. Scheider, MD, and colleagues at the University of Cincinnati, says groups with the highest risk and frequency of stroke, such as people over 75 years old, blacks, and men, were the least knowledgeable about stroke warning signs and risk factors. According to several national organizations, major warning signs of stroke include:

- Sudden numbness or weakness of the face, arm, or leg – especially on one side of the body
- Sudden confusion or trouble speaking or understanding speech
- Sudden trouble seeing in one or both eyes
- Sudden trouble walking, dizziness, or loss of balance or coordination
- Sudden, severe headache that comes on with no known cause

Factors that are known to increase a person's risk of suffering a stroke include:
- High blood pressure

- Smoking
- Heart disease
- Diabetes
- History of stroke or transient ischemic attack (also known as mini-stroke)
- Heavy alcohol use
- High cholesterol levels

I have none of those. Although my grandparents lived at younger, failing to make a life at an older age. I know that I must be willing to have a middle life, correct? But among four grandparents, suppose they are dying a fire, or died accidentally by a car or maybe they were (and it was that unusual) to die from the flu or even pneumonia. Or, for example, even our family was heavy drinkers, if they were totally lushes? It's bad for me? Since my grandparents (except one grandmother and my mother who is 85) were died before 60? Again, it's bad for me? There are problems and they are not inherited.

Researchers found people most frequently cited television, magazines and daily newspapers as their source of knowledge about stroke. But in light of these findings, some of them false, the study researchers said that public education efforts must continue and should focus on groups at the highest risk of stroke. A TIA (transient ischemic attack) signals trouble in the arteries bringing the oxygen, sugar, and other nutrients to its brain, causing a temporary blockage of an artery. When lacking blood flow is caused by a clot, it can be brief or even minor. A momentary clot will prepare the loss of function to a normal, blood flow that can be restored. These attacks indicate that something is wrong and tell you of a warning of a stroke.

At a medical conference on strokes, they didn't say much about drug therapy. Many textbooks write about speech therapy, it does not mention about drugs. It seemed like medicine does not articulate speech therapy. The opposite of medical classes don't have speech and communication classes. Speech and language is a part of journalism and public affairs. There are two different strategies, two different environments. They are even different buildings and opposite from campuses. There is not a chance of two spheres or two orbits crashing. Doctors give you a speech therapist and their hands are cleaned. You are repaired from a stroke; let the speech or occupational therapists get along with the patient. "Opponents objected that this type of research was arid and superficial, neither interesting nor generizable to the complex conditions of human interactions," said *The Broken Brain, the Biological Revolution in Psychiatry* from Nancy Andreasen, MD, PhD. In medical jargon, "Psychiatrists, who were becoming principally psychoanalytically oriented, rarely bothered to pay close attention to behavioral theories and research; when they did, they frequently objected that the work of the behaviorists was of little help in understanding abnormal behavior and that its 'black box' approach was mechanistic, oversimplified, and even inhumane."

Still, my speech therapist will ask, "What color is the fire engine?" Blue, maybe. Black? I didn't like my therapist. I heard the question, and I was angry. What color is the grass? What color, Ms. Speech Therapist, you've been smoking grass? What color is it? Green, maybe? Don't belittle me. Don't talk with me as you would want to talk with a 5-year-old child. I finished grade school, thank you. Explain to the patients or ask them or test them what they are: their brains or their intellectual powers had accidents, and were fragile. Don't take a lot of time with learning either you or I. My bills are outrageous, even paying with health insurance. I'm still paying with bills charged from speech therapists two years after my stroke. My time has been limited. I didn't want to go to speech therapy after a year. It was fine six weeks or six months pre-stroke, but after a year it was too long, too expensive, and my results were too unsatisfactory. An additional 2.6 million people between ages of 18-64, were uninsured for more than a year. Who can blame them keeping speech therapy after two years or five years for a stroke?

Blaming the brain

Elliot Valenstein, PhD, a neurologist from the University of Michigan, had a theory of drug action and biochemical causes of mental disorder, in the "Blaming the Brain; the Truth About Drugs and Mental Health." Velenstein wrote: "The claim that drugs could treat mental disorders was initially met with considerable skepticism. Many psychiatrists found it difficult to believe that a drug could remove the repressed conflicts that were thought to underlie most mental disorders." It was concluded that drugs might temporarily loosen certain symptoms. They would soon be replaced by other symptoms. "Most psychiatrists believed that patients had to be made aware of their unconscious fears, desires, and conflicts" before any lasting help could be achieved and this could be accomplished within the case of psychotherapy. Although his book in about mental disorder he mentions Zoloft, a few of the psychoactive drugs that are calmed with patients from a stroke. "You know when you're not feeling like yourself," reads Zoloft advertising. "You're tired all the time. You may feel sad, hopeless – and lose interest in things you once loved. You may feel anxious and can't even sleep. Your daily activities and relationships suffer." The depression means restlessness or slowed movements, fatigue or lack of energy, changes in appetite or weight, feeling worthless or guilty for no real reason, trouble concentrating or making decisions, and repeated thoughts of death of suicide. Panic disorder is a fast heart rate or pounding heart, chest pain or discomfort, sweating, trembling or shaking, shortness of breath or a feeling of smothering, choking feeling, etc. Zoloft is not for everyone. The most common ones are dry mouth, diarrhea/loose stools, feeling unusually tired or sleepy, trouble sleeping, sexual problems in men and women, tremor, etc. Everyone has a normal substance in the brain called serotonin. It is thought that not having enough serotonin may contribute to depression, panic disorder, obsessive compulsive disorder and posttraumatic stress disorder. Prozac, Luvox and Pavil are others pyschoceutical, a sort of a link between treatments for patients who are at risk for heart problems. They are SSRIs (selective serontonin reuptake inhibitors). Whether lowered platelets translates to reduced heart diseases and stroke, some agree. However, they can be too strong to prescribe to healthy people. I don't take Zoloft. I am not depressed even after I was losing my job and my wife. I really am not depressed, I'm just unlucky! DO NOT take drugs if you're not certain what they do, and what your symptoms are. A lot of intelligent people have said that to me. I believe that. But, depression can significantly increase a heart attack and stroke survivor's chances of a second episode, reports stated. Depression alters:

- Cardiac rhythms
- Increases blood pressure
- Raises insulin levels

"Mental illness" is a way of drugs that cause the stroke patients from a soothing and milder stress, and easier of an impending attack. The relentless exposure to daily, chronic anxiety is the most toxic form of stress. Researchers have tied stress resistance to a bundle of coping strategies described by one word: resilience. Those who handle stress well recover quickly, physically and mentally, when faced with it. Train yourself to deal with stress everyday.

"Traumatic life events" is about the issue in Assessment and Management of Emotional and Psychosocial Reactions to Brain Damage and Aphasia by Peter Wahrborg. Depressed was a study seen as two years from a stroke. Insomnia, eating (or not eating), fatigue, etc. are all be plainly seen. The obvious that each male sees to have his own threshold for psychosomatic reactions and his own combination of stress variables. They are:

- The duration of the stress needed to activate a warning symptom can vary.
- The frequency of stress experiences that can be tolerated can vary.
- The intensity of the stress as it is subjectively experienced is different for each man and can influence the appearance of a stress symptom.

- The confluence or sequence of stresses can lead to different stress outcomes. If the death of a parent precedes a minor accident, the victim may feel far more anxious and dependent than he would, had the preceding stress been assuming a larger mortgage!
- The symbolic meaning of a particular stress to a particular person can affect its stress impact.

According to *The Male Stress Survival Guide* by Georgia Wikin, PhD, "Early warning signals, then, not only help men to head off the more serious consequence of male stress, but also can help men learn about their own emotional learning history, their own readiness to cope or capitulate to particular stresses, their own symptom patterns, their own psychological and physical vulnerabilities, and their own personality profiles."

From a National Aphasia Association newsletter, it writes about aphasia and medicine: "Aphasia Therapy in the New Millennium" by Kristine Lundgren and Martin L. Albert. I wondered if there were no drugs for prescribed aphasia. Therapy seemed to be belonged to synonyms, morphemic usage, and sentence construction. That's really good, but that's not really prescribing or even describing drugs, are they? They are few at mentions, or even none, at reading textbooks for aphasia. A random book's index does not have any terms of biotechnology, drugs, and constraint-induced therapy. "Pharmacological approaches to aphasia continue to generate excitement," said in the newsletter about strokes. In a study used cholinergic (neurotransmitter) therapy. This therapy involves using drugs to improve the functioning of the damaged brain. It sounded like a better method. Many of my speech therapists don't even have a clue about drugs vs. aphasia, or about Aricept or about transcranial magnetic stimulation (TMS). They will say, "Ask your doctor" or "ask your pharmacist." Should our speech therapists, who will work with their patients with hours or weeks or months, tell us about their questions? They don't understand neurons, the brain or drugs. They know words or sentences. They aren't medical personnel or doctors. Doctors don't know words or sentences (or even patients, but that's another thing!)

The other ones used a different neurotransmitter, bromocriptine (a dopaminergic agent) combined the speech therapy. But never imagine a neurologist recommending bromocriptine with patients for their speech problems. Or the opposite: a speech pathologist giving the patient a listing of word power with a study of proteomics. It's a problem with our words: medicine vs. communication. It's a matter of electricity and mechanical vs. biology and anatomy. I don't expect them to understand everything, but I do expect them to communicate or understand each field. I am a patient with a ping pong ball. Back and forth, back and forth. Around and around. Their results found that drugs, that is bromocriptine, improved the verbal performance of the subject. Of the use of amphetamines was also featured to treat aphasia. They found amphetamines paired with regular speech/language therapy facilitated language recovery in the period shortly after stroke. They didn't know. I had frustration, a feeling of disappointed with my aphasia.

Piracetam has been tested on patients with aphasia in several clinical research trials in Germany. It holds promise for treatment of aphasia. Results from studies using pharmacologic interventions for the treatment of aphasia have been encouraging. Dextroamphetamine (Dexedrine trademark) improves attention span and enhances learning and memory.

Researchers are also looking at nontraditional treatments, i.e. "constraint-induced (CI) therapy" to treat language disorders in subjects with chronic aphasia. This approach was used originally in subjects, i.e., paralysis of an arm or a leg following a stroke. In patients with aphasia, the same test applied: constraint-induced therapy requires that a patient in intensive practice of one means of expression (speaking out loud) while restricting the use of alternative methods (gesturing). With this technique, the authors found significant improvements in the ability of a small group of patients with chronic aphasia to verbalize in a relatively short period.

Psychological factors may indirectly address a therapy. Laura Murray and her colleagues "used relaxation therapy in conjunction with traditional aphasia therapy to improve verbal performance in chronic nonfluent aphasic subjects." Relaxation training included both guided imagery and progressive muscle relaxation. It can only train with a nonfluent aphasia. During the past two years, a therapist decided which techniques to use and to give, accordingly, to the patient.

The knowledge of attention theory may influence the evaluation and treatment of language production and comprehension in adults with aphasia. If an individual has difficulty with attention, that fact may negatively affect any types of speech and language therapy. These researchers compared two widely used techniques. "Context-based" or a specific context or a casual conversation, and a "skill-based" treatment in which the specific tasks needed to improve oral reading. A skill-based treatment has an impact on the individual use of a language than context-based treatment.

Advances in research on neural regeneration and the use of biotechnology will also influence the future of aphasia therapy. And the field of brain cell transplantation is still in its infancy and is fraught with controversy, but represents a direction to watch over the next few years.

In the field of biotechnology, repetitive transcranial magnetic stimulation (TMI or rTMS) has been used on a small group of patients with nonfluent aphasia to improve naming skills. The researchers at Aphasia Research Center at Boston University School of Medicine and from Boston's Beth Israel Deaconess Medical Center and Harvard Medical School used some possibilities with magnetic stimulation to influence brain function in various regions of the brain cortex. So far, this response has a small group of subjects, and highly experimental, but has demonstrated improvement in the field for nonfluent (not articulate) patients.

With the responses of the patients, it is important to have small quantity of individuals. However, "We continue to hope that research of this type will yield successful therapy techniques for individuals with aphasia." Aphasia research is exploring new ways to evaluate and treat aphasia as well as to further understanding of the function of the brain. Biotech and bioscience are hoping, at least for now. Their ability to apply research progress in clinical practice stimulates the development of a large number of drugs and innovations.

Neurologist: drugs aren't simple

A neurologist tells me, no drugs are simple and they don't always work. Take time to understand your drugs. Drugs are expensive, and some drugs are dangerous or don't work or if they're inaccurately or mistakenly prescribed. Speech therapy is cheaper (relatively), and is primarily paid by insurance (for example, 80% paid by health insurance). In speech therapy, 10 years they were still using a Language Master machine. You would feed the cards in them, like an old-fashioned, early computer. That is a long time ago when you think about it. The computers were very fast, had mega-memory, had extra accessories, etc. in the last decade. "In the future, we may be certain that dramatic progress will continue in the development and application of scientific aids to speech therapy," wrote David Knox, "Portrait of Aphasia." It was written in 1985. That Hewitt Packard computer, with the Win95 word software, and has given me for my occupation. I am an old geezer. That was an old, old computer. I got since then Windows, Win98 and 2001, Microsoft Office, Excel, Internet and emails. I thought about my speech classes and my training from the ancient Language Master, oh supreme being! It reminds me of the old cartoon Felix the Cat and his antagonist. I remembered he had sort of an evil face with black eyes, arms with hooks not hands, without legs named the Master Cylinder. The Master Cylinder or the Language Master should be... canned.

An aspirin is an almost-free drug, and is by almost preferred from medical doctors. A penny for an aspirin – that is one of our best generics. One theory doesn't like taking or prescribing aspirin. A researcher says exercise and a regular diet may be some help in place of aspirin. I am fortunate in that I can exercise and run or bicycle. I can bike from my condo to the library. I got a backpack for books and magazines and videos. I can carry a gallon of milk and a half-gallon orange juice with my bike from the grocery store! It's not easy, but I can carry a lot. Carrying in my back, carrying in my bike rack – it's almost easier than driving my van or my car in traffic. It's nice to biking in spring or summer or fall days. But not everyone can exercise or they can't exercise intensely because of high blood pressure. My pressure is always near 120. Mild elevations are around 140/90 to 159/94. Many must restrict salt and desist smoking cigarettes. Incidentally, "low tar" cigarettes are as much harmful as other cigarettes. People who switch to low-tar or light cigarettes are likely to inhale the same amount of cancer-causing toxins. Those smokers face a high risk of cancer and other diseases from tar and other toxins. Many people have high blood pressure are too fat. They must lose extra pounds.

Another researcher said we have taught too little as a means of explaining strokes. Charles Warlow in England received his medical training at Cambridge University and then St George's Hospital Medical School in London. He began in 1971 where he started his research into stroke. He then trained in neurology. Warlow established his reputation in stroke research. Since then he has built up a team of senior clinical researchers into many aspects of stroke. He also has research interests in motor neurons disease, intracranial vascular malformations and medically unexplained symptoms.

Warlow told researchers and medical personnel, evaluating treatments in stroke is too slow. I agree with Warlow's research. It was time to get out of the second gear, or within the second century. "We have had in our hands for over half a century a remarkable tool to evaluate therapeutic interventions, the randomized controlled trial," he said. "And we have had meta-analysis for two decades. But it still generally takes us far too long to assess treatments for acute stroke, and for stroke rehabilitation, and to prevent recurrence."

We are a disappearance, the bridge that is broken. A medical textbook does not appear speech therapy. You talk to a neurologist. The neurologist said there's nothing wrong, since the patient is still standing, his heart is still beating. You'll keep talking, but the neurologist only says if when, where and time is there. A patient can yell, "Fire!" If you're physically nothing wrong, then you should see a speech therapist or psychiatrist – with no drugs, or other response. There is no single reason for this tardiness, Warlow said. The difficulties in stroke certainly include doctor ignorance. Generic difficulties include the tedium of some randomized trials, their length and their cost, the lack of credit for collaborating in them, and the increasing height and number of hurdles erected in our path by ethicists

Slow progress has been made. They were they were haphazard – stroke units, aspirin, anticoagulants, carotid surgery, long term blood pressure and cholesterol lowering. An easier-to-use blood thinner pill offers the first potential alternative from warfarin in more than 50 years. The standard treatment given to millions of people can prevent blood clots. It prevents clot by acting more quickly and does not require the frequent blood testing of Coumadin, a brand name for warfarin. It is widely prescribed after strokes but also heart attacks and other orthopedic surgery like knee replacements, to recur clots in legs or lungs. Heparin was among the anticoagulants. Often, effective action can often returns a stroke victim to normal. An exercise, an aspirin daily, and a low-cholesterol diet can prescribe any patient, without even handling a speech therapy. Various surgeries can clear out obstructions in their blood vessels. Perhaps the quickest was one of the most recent which is optimism is coiling rather than clipping intracranial aneurysms. These advances have all improved. Four blood clots are mentioned: the stationary clot in the brain and heart. Traveling clot which comes developed in the heart of blood vessels, remaining at the brain. A similar bleeding artery, which causes a weakness in the blood walls of a brain and a weakness in the lower brain, called an aneurysm.

"In the future, our trials should address sensible questions that haven't already been answered," Warlow said. "They should exploit the uncertainty principle to combine best science with best ethics, they should be simple but not simple-minded, they should be inexpensive, and they should be part of the routine business of clinical medicine. It helps to have more than one trial running simultaneously, and independent of any sponsors. Trials should also be educational for the collaborators, fun too but still deadly serious. Then we may get the evidence we need to change practice much faster. So let's get into third gear and even dream about top gear and the open road ahead!"

Change our practices, make them faster – that's a speedy, 100 miles per hour! Let's go full-time ahead...

Educate the public

The NAA's mission is "to educate the public to know that the word aphasia describes an impairment of the ability to communicate, not an impairment of intellect. The NAA makes people with aphasia, their families, support systems, and health care professionals aware of resources to recover lost skills to the extent possible, to compensate for skills that will not be recovered and to minimize the psychosocial impact of the language impairment."

The Stroke Council web site gives the role of warfarin (pronounced WAR-far-in) as the primary or secondary stroke prevention, with not much future. Warfarin (brand name "Coumadin") is not superior to aspirin for preventing a second stroke for patients. A non-cardioembolic stroke reported in the Warfarin-Aspirin Recurrent Stroke Study (WARSS). The primary endpoint of the WARSS trial was recurrent stroke or death from any cause within two years of blinded treatment with warfarin or aspirin or taking daily "baby"aspirin (lower than 75 mg). WARSS found no significant difference between the two treatment groups in recurrent ischemic stroke, death, or serious hemorrhage. Even in cases of so called "aspirin failure", patients who had a stroke while taking aspirin before entering the study, warfarin was no better than taking daily aspirin in preventing recurrent stroke. For prevention of secondary stroke for patients with normal heart function and rhythm, warfarin given to achieve any INR level is more costly and difficult to manage than aspirin. There are new and novel drugs compared to warfarin.

An anticoagulant has possible side effects:
- Bleeding from the gums or nose
- Coughing up blood
- Red or black bowel movements
- Red or dark-brown colored urine
- Unusually heavy menstrual bleeding
- Heavy bleeding from cuts or wounds that does not stop
- Easy bruising, purple spots on the skin
- Severe headache

If you have problems with less serious side effects such as loss of appetite, mild stomach cramps, or upset stomach, tell your doctor.

It is very important to have regular blood tests done while taking warfarin to determine the proper and safe dose. It is common while taking this medicine to have your dose changed. You should carry an identification card that shows that you are taking warfarin or taking any blood-thinner drugs.

It's a real boon to aspirin. It's inexpensive (cheap) and generic. But it doesn't always be safer or sound. Warfarin remains the treatment of choice for patients with nonvalvular atrial fibrillation (NVAF) with prior TIA or stroke. Patients can take it safely and for selected NVAF high risk patients for primary prevention. As well as patients with higher risk of cerebral embolization associated with a cardiac valvular prosthesis constructed of synthetic materials. Patients with NVAF who take warfarin to achieve an INR range of 2.0 - 3.0 have stroke reduced by 65% versus no antithrombotic therapy and by 45% compared to aspirin treatment. Ongoing prospective trials compared warfarin to aspirin in other disorders with increased stroke risk, described by the Stroke Trials Directory web site.

Until these studies are completed and published, the current data support aspirin and/or other antiplatelet agents, rather than warfarin, as treatments of choice for most patients to prevent recurrent non-cardioembolic stroke.

A researcher, Peter Libby, MD, cardiovascular medicine, said aspirin and an inflammatory response doesn't always have a chance – at aspirin means as little as 2 cents per tablet, or $2 for a 100-aspirin bottle from the everyday corner drug store. "Contrary to public perception, the heart attacks and strokes that result from this condition exceed cancer as a cause of death in industrial nations and are growing more prevalent in developing countries as well." Libby said the problem is plaque and a thrombus. Looking into a microscopic blood clots, "some clots dissolve before they cause a heart attack or stroke, but they can foster trouble in another way – by stimulating plaque expansion... Our bodies produce substances that can prevent a clot from materializing or can degrade it before it causes a heart attack or stroke, but inflamed plaques release chemicals that impede the innate clot-busting machinery." A lifestyle modification as cardiovascular prevention by modifying diet and recommended exercise, like running or biking, playing tennis or golfing.

Researchers are working a stroke damage, a contrarian to Warlow. Scientists working with mice have found that a compound used to fight severe blood infections may be useful in preventing stroke damage. Activated protein C was found to reduce the likelihood that brain cells would self-destruct after a stroke, the researchers reported in the journal *Nature Medicine*. "Strokes occur when the blood supply is cut off to part of the brain, by a blood clot for example. Some cells die right away; others are damaged and self-destruct later in a process called apoptosis." When mice had a stroke, some 65% of the cells that would have died after the stroke survived. The mice treated with the protein.

The protein also is the active ingredient in a drug approved for human use in the treatment of sepsis, a severe blood infection that can be deadly. In that case it acts by reducing blood clotting and inflammation. After a stroke victim, the protein decreases the cellular signals that persuade brain cells to kill themselves after a stroke and boost signals that persuade the cells to survive.

The heart, aorta, and major arteries in the head and neck are the usual places where clots or other particles break loose and travel to arteries in the brain, called a brain infarct or a stroke. The blood infiltrates into the brain under pressure and forms a localized, often round or elliptical blood, known as a hematoma. The bleeding into the left cerebral hemisphere, can often leave a weakness and loss of the feeling in the right limbs and loss of normal speech.

A report also that injury to blood vessels during angioplasty, a vessel clearing procedure, can lead to proliferation of vessel cells and renewed blockage. This complication occurs in almost a third of patients, who often must undergo repeat angioplasties. A single, one-hour treatment of carbon monoxide given to rats can cut down on the long-term damage to vessels after angioplasty.

Researchers found that low levels of carbon monoxide increased of the smooth muscle cells that form the vessel walls. A long-term administration of carbon monoxide reduced the arteriosclerotic lesions caused by transplantation. It was a problem that occurs in people caused an organ rejection after vessel grafting. It's known that a carbon monoxide-producing enzyme in the body protects against vessel injury from transplantation. But it's unclear whether carbon monoxide could exert such effects direct. In 1975-86, the death rate from stroke declined a remarkable 33%.

What is your cholesterol?

A person's body hovered around 170/100 mg/dl of cholesterol. Do you have a high cholesterol lifestyle? My cholesterol is 207 mg/dl. If you have any heart disease or stroke, 190 or more cholesterol after three months of diet changes, the physician may prescribe 160-189 LDL. Your LDL goal is before 160. With two or more risk factors other than high LDL cholesterol, your 10-year risk of heart disease is 20% or less. One hundred sixty or more after three months of diets may prescribe sooner. The LDL goal is less than 130. Not every person whose cholesterol is between 200 and 239 mg/dl is at increased risk for developing atherosclerosis. This increases their total cholesterol. Trust your doctor to interpret your results.

Everyone's case is different. If your cholesterol is over 240, it's definitely high. Your risk of heart attack or stroke is greater and you need more tests. The chances are:

• You buy a lot of prepared convenience, and fast food. If you (like most) can eat a quick meal for lunch, it means a burger-fries-coke.

• You eat a lot of fried or breaded food. You get meals with a bun for driving in your car.

• You've been putting off losing those extra pounds. I weighed 160 pounds for a job that had at a computer and phone for eight hours. After eight hours I was too tired and too hungry for an hour at the YMCA. There was no time, plenty of excuses. I was just too tired for exercise.

• You've never had your cholesterol level checked – or for five years or more.

There's more. Here is a guide to low-cholesterol living:
• Limit to three eggs per week (french toast is about 1 egg with two slices).

• Limit (or even absent) pork (the alternative white meat). Delete bacon, sausage, and fatty fowls (duck and goose), skin and fat of turkey and chicken; luncheon meats such as salami and baloney); hot dogs; tuna in oil; kidneys and liver. Shellfish (lobster, shrimp, crab, oysters), a dinner can be sparingly eaten.

• Avoid avocados and olives. Starchy vegetables from potatoes, corn, lima beans – ok, if they're substituting for a serving of bread or cereal.

• Avoid baked goods; donuts, sweet rolls, cakes and pies (you know that!).

• Avoid whole milk; ice cream; yogurt or cheese.

• Avoid nuts; pecans, walnuts and peanuts to limited one tablespoonful per day.

• Snack on air-popped popcorn, low-salt pretzels.

• Dinner: have spaghetti with tomato sauce, also turkey breast lean meatballs.

Polyunsaturated and monounsaturated fatty acids are the two unsaturated fatty acids. They're often found in liquid oils from plants. Common sources of polyunsaturated fatty acids are safflower, sesame and sunflower seeds, corn and soybeans, many nuts and seeds, and their oils. Canola, olive and peanut oils, and avocados are sources of monounsaturated fatty acids. American Heart Association said that your polyunsaturated fatty acid intake should be up to 10% of total calories, and up to 15% of total calories, made up monounsaturated fatty acids. Margarine should be limited. It's better than fats with a high saturated fatty acid content, such as butter, lard or hydrogenated shortenings.

Atherosclerosis is a process by which fatty deposits accumulate and build up on the inner lining of the arteries. Fats dissolved in the blood may precipitate out of solution faster in the presence of prolonged elevated blood pressure. Atherosclerosis is the hardening of the walls of the arteries, making them less elastic and endure perhaps cushioning the higher systolic pressures generated by the heart (can lead to a stroke). The greater the duration of stress, the longer the increase in blood pressure; the longer the increase in blood pressure, the greater the amount of fatty deposits (cholesterol). It's known as the "cholesterol connection."

You need regular checkups to monitor blood pressure changes, cardiac irregularities, and digestive problems to assess the cause of backaches and headaches. Diagnose chronic fatigue, hyperventilation, muscle spasm, chest pains, dizziness, cold sweats, nausea and increased allergies reactions. You may also need to monitor signs of diseases and disorders that are not caused or aggravated by stress.

The Centocor Company had developed ReoPro, a protein on the surface of platelets, which promote the formation of blood clots. By preventing platelets from sticking, it reduces the chance of lethal clot formation patients undergoing angioplasty. Biotech companies are interested in cloning genes with protein products. Receptors often belong to large families of similar proteins. A drug may indeed effectively target a receptor relevant to the disease in question. Among the most eagerly sought are the genes for proteins usually found on cell surfaces that serve as receptors for neutrotransmitters, hormones and growth factors. Statins alone reduce a person's heart disease risk by 25% to 30%. New studies find that the drugs lower the risk of stroke and heart attacks in people at high risk for heart disease but whose cholesterol levels may be normal of even low. Statins can pose dangers to some people more than others. Statins block the formation of cholesterol. They have health risks of their own. It's clear that statin therapy alone isn't enough. A protein called Apo A-1 Milano is a version of HDL, a good cholesterol, which loads fats from arteries. Statins block the production of low-density lipoprotein (LDL), or bad cholesterol. High-dose therapy with niacin, now offered in time-release form, offers some benefit, but many people shrink from the side effects, which including facial heat and redness.

St. John Macomb Hospital Medical Director of Cardiovascular Services, Lingareddy Devireddy, said that heart attacks can be further treated by administering clot busting medicine that dissolves the blockage. "With this form of therapy, there is a 1-2% risk of developing a stroke. The risk of stroke is even higher in those over the age of 75."

Very low-density lipoprotein (VLDL), low-density lipoprotein (LDL), and high-density lipoproten (HDL). VLDL carries fats to different parts of the body; HDL returns cholesterol left in the blood vessels to the liver; LDL carries cholesterol to different parts of the body. HDLs pick up stuck cholesterol and bring them back to the liver. If more cholesterol is leaving in the blood vessels, HDLs can't flush them. If this happens in a blood vessel in your heart, a heart attack may result. Some people have a genetic problem. They are born with a "liver warehouse" that simply makes too much cholesterol and therefore has too many LDLs. Early in life we all start to develop plaque (including cholesterol) along the arterial walls throughout our bodies. If a clot forms in an artery supplying the heart, a heart attack can occur. If a clot forms in an artery supplying the brain, it can result in a stroke.

There are 800,000 heart attacks each year in the United States; 213,000 are fatals – quite a lot, more than 25%. Angioplasty, referred to the balloon, is the preferred strategy to restore blood flow. Drug-stents are used to support the artery and reduce the chance of recurrence of the blockage, which became operational in early 2003. The Cypher stent is coated with a drug to stop the growth of unwanted tissue from plugging up the blood vessel. Cypher is in the bare-metal stent. It contributed to a decline in bypass surgery. Cardiologists say drug coatings make angioplasty nearly as reliable as a bypass operation, replacing the two-week recovery time with after the operation. Similarly non-invasive procedures will fix heart valves and to prevent stroke by clearing plaque from the carotid arteries, which supply blood to the brain. Angioplasty offers a quicker recovery than bypass surgery. The doctor works through a small opening in the femoral artery in the groin, not an eight- to 10-inch incision in the chest. The doctor guides a tiny balloon to a blockage near the heart and clears the clog by inflating the balloon. The balloon simultaneously expands the stent, opening the artery.

The "beta-blockers" are researched with Zocor (trademark) made by Merck and Pravachol (trademark) by Bristol-Myers Squibb. "Even if you are totally dedicated to your diet and exercise program, you may need to add Zocor to your routine to reach a healthy cholesterol level" said an ad. In national newspapers, Bristol-Myers Squibb advertised: "Pravachol is the only cholesterol lowering drug proven to help prevent first and second heart attack and stroke in people with high cholesterol or heart disease." This suggested that Pravachol proved to help prevent stroke in people without heart disease. Pravachol has not been proven to help prevent strokes without heart disease. It is proven to aid preventing stroke only in people with coronary heart disease. Pravachol is still a better choice for heart disease.

Smarter treatments

Our new understanding of fear has also generated smarter pharmacological treatments for post-traumatic stress disorder. They are two recent studies that involved giving beta-blockers to patients in a stressful life, who has recently suffered a traumatic event. They can play a direct role in life-and-death struggles. It's not surprising to find that the brain contains elaborate machinery assigned to its routines. That emotional excitement triggers the memory-enhancing cycle all over again, making the traumatic memory-enhancing cycle all over again, making the traumatic memory even stronger. "By preventing the autonomic reaction beta-blockers keep the memory from forming deeper grooves in the brain, making post-traumatic stress symptoms less severe," said a Discover magazine (March 2003). The National Cholesterol Education Program states your doctor should prescribe an anti-cholesterol with the patient, over 200 mg/dl include:

Cigarette smoking
Overweight
Heart disease
Diabetes
Over 45 age for a man, or a woman over 55
A family of early heart disease

The population is people with limits of cholesterol at least 50% of all people. At a seminar for public meetings, lecturing from the cardiovascular doctor of St. John Hospital, the middle or older population is become an aging and smarter for the medical users – not necessarily patients. They have a chance to ask a question, when they are not thinking of it when they are at a physical exam. Most are intelligent to set their cholesterol goal, reduce their heart risks, and change their diets.

I've always liked a glass of red wine. That's my favorite prescription. But only once daily, not twice or three times! If you drink them, do so in moderation. If your vision is too blurring and your language is too slurry, obviously you're drinking too much! Have no more than one drink per day (for women) or two drinks per day (for men) of wine, beer or liquor. "People who have more than two alcoholic drinks per day on an ongoing basis have a tenfold increased risk of a subarachnoid hemorrhage stroke," according to Blue Cross Blue Shield. Usually painful and devastating, these stroke occur at an average age of about 50, and nearly 40% of those who suffer them die within 30 days, according to the American Stroke Association. Drinking alcohol is a drug. Moderation is a good limit.

Chapter 7

Marriage and jobs: one plus one equal stress

Maybe when you die, you come before a big bearded man on a big throne, and you say, "Is this heaven?" And he says, "Heaven? You just came from there."
Kirk Douglas

Those two significant changes with aphasia are:

Your job. It won't be. Your job has not something originally you have. "Your job" maybe isn't the same, means something different. It means that somebody else takes your job. You didn't have "your job." You had a career, it can be done at anyone. It's one that you had – maybe a year, 10 years, even 20 years. You did the work and it means you made it differently, right or wrong. Part of communications in the workplace can be relevant to persons with aphasia. Get *The Legal Aspects of Aphasia,* a 23-page report by the American Bar Association in 1983, phone 800-922-4622. The American with Disabilities (ADA) ensures access to public transit and places of business. To obtain a copy, phone 301-897-5700 or write American Speech-Language Hearing Association (ASHA), Director of Multicultural Resource Services, 10801 Rockville Pike, Rockville, MD 20852. "There is more likelihood of clients in this group wishing to return to work, though only a percentage of them will be able to, and many of these may well need to return to a modified form of employment. For the majority, early retirement is the most likely option," from "Working With Apraxic Clients."

Early retirement is an option? Is it a preference or only the alternative? The Riley Guide, www.rileyguide.com is a nifty Internet with more than 13,000 sites devoted to some aspect of up-to-date jobs.

Divorce – look up for anxiety and apprehension. Tension. Look up at the description of stress. In Merriam Webster's dictionary there are 16 lines under "stress." It said, physical, chemical and emotional caused by a bodily or mental force. The death of a spouse is a number termed "100" for a life change index scale drawn by Thomas Holmes. A divorce was termed 73, rating at the second of the scale. Death of a close family is "only" 53, being fired at work is a 45. By interpreting your score, 300 or above, creates a major life crisis level with an 80% chance of illness. My scale is about 5,000, I think. I thought about my life. "Success in managing stress will not come overnight, and it will not come at all if approached half-heartedly. It will take determination, persistence and time, but the results will be well worth the effort," says *Divorce and Beyond*, by James Greteman and Leon Haverkamp. They have a mask to cover up our anger. Actor: creates scenes; quick tempered; hot headed. The blamer: throws away responsibility for the way they act or feel toward others. I have my own category. The aphasic: can't tell his ex-wife how he is angry and depressed with her, and cold or distant from her. When asked, "What is the good and bad of your stroke?" it's simple – the good/bad from me is divorce and retirement. It was good, and bad, both simultaneously divorce and retirement.

Jobs

To get a job and keep the bosses happy include:
• To help ensure that the organization is able to attract, retain and motivate the caliber of individuals necessary to achieve the organization's goals. Don't be an anchor.
• To remain competitive in the labor market for comparable jobs (the external factor). Positions and salary ranges are reviewed from time to time to determine competitiveness.

- Maintain equity in the relationship of pay within the organization (internal factor).
- To pay and reward superior levels of performance.
- To comply with all government regulations and ensure fair treatment of all employees regardless of race, color, sex, religion, age, national origin, handicap or any other basis made illegal by applicable law.

I was time to adjust retiring. I was not really retiring at before 50. I was just tipping one toe in the bathtub of workplace. I was to attend at a contractors' and engineers' meeting at a national heating and air conditioning convention. I was not attending at Business News Publishing trade magazine's reporter or editor or publisher, but I was there at an independent freelance media credentials. I was proud to have a press badge. It was a cheap plastic badge with my name on it. It showed to everyone a Purple Heart medal. My credentials were convincing and competent, I thought. I was still alive! It was surprising to see my former employees, manufacturers, exhibitors and contractors. I was sort of not talking, just nodding my head, walking and saying "Good to see you," and say hi and bye. Take technical papers at the meeting afterward. Hear a few words for seminars and symposiums. I avoided long conversations. I couldn't speak too many sentences. I was aphasic. I sought as a freelancing writer. I drove from Detroit to Chicago, with maps printed on my computer, to drive Chicago's McCormick Place Convention. I drove alone, 270 miles one way, 540 miles away in one day. It was cheaper from after my retirement wages. I didn't have an expense account. During my career, I was a publisher on an excellent trade magazine. The readers loved it. We were kind of a tool: the magazine was reference manual, news of their interest, a social and human interest of feature articles. The magazine was 65 years old. My company bought it a few years ago. The readers still were interested in my magazine. Circulation was strong, and advertisers were happy to spend their ads in my pages. We were partners with our readers. We were a combination of contractors and journalists in a trade magazine.

Driving with the King

"Before you try to drive, get clearance from your doctor," reminds of a book on stroke. "If your doctor says it's okay for you to drive, contact your State Department of Motor Vehicles and ask which requirements apply to you. It's possible you'll have to take a new road test..." Three days from getting a stroke, I was not able to drive a car. The doctor or the department of motor vehicles didn't get my ok for my driving. They didn't allow me, nor given me a test. Ask yourself: can I drive ok? Can I have accidents driving my car? I was careful. Tell that to a drunk. There isn't approval or permission or sanctimony. You have the King waiting. He is a passenger. You're the only one there in the driver's seat. I had no accidents and no tickets from my days of my stroke, driving two years plus. Knock on wood.

Marriage

It's time for meeting a support group, that means a divorce workshop. That is a wrong idea. Divorce is a bad word. It means – well, it means *divorce:* dead end or disappearing or denial of marriage. As a sudden tragic or despair from yourself. Some people don't even like the word, divorce. They'll talk about parting the ways, or a separation of maintenance. A support group is there to help you. They will help you and aid you, where the divorce seems an end or a dead life. They will try to or support you to feel a life, a lifestyle. I thought about a divorce. It's a long maze, not an extinct life. There is an extended life. You are in it, and you crash in the brick wall. A workshop is similar to aphasia. It sounds so grim! The walking, a wheelchair or cane is helping patients for a stroke. But beware of the difficult emotions without helping the participants. Aphasia is also a long maze. There is an extended life, not extinction. It doesn't suddenly "broke up" or "failed" the marriage. The marriage ended, that's all. It ended, and put in a period. Divorce means denial, deception, disappear, dire (exciting, horror!), a dirge –

a song or hymn of grief or lamentation. It doesn't disappear. Why deception accompanies a divorce? Get along with your divorce and put the period after it.

Jobs + marriage = stress

A social-psychological book includes the subject "stress" for its chapter. One of the primary contributors to stress is anxiety. Another contributor addressing stress is the phenomenon known as the 'flooding of emotions.' Stress is a metaphor for stroke. One of the contributors to stroke is anxiety also. Yet another stroke factor is being overloaded. There are things to do and too little time. Stroke means stress. Divorcing people need to keep their freedom from disease, to have enough energy to take control of their present lives. If stress can cause physical illness, all the way from headaches to heart attacks can be introduced.

Share your experiences, thoughts and feelings openly. I thought it was just talking in interviews with authors selling another best seller, or among psychiatrists. I didn't think it was a disease. Consider it for genuine. Express your feelings and don't be afraid to open your worst feelings. Respect and accept each other in the group for what and who they are. Help others to explore and developing ideas and feelings they are giving them too. (No hustling is another no-no we were told. "We are not here as a dating service." Well, I'm sorry but I am very happy to feel or understand to someone, maybe a woman. They can be a shoulder to cry on, and help is not just a duty. Seminars are divorce workshops – of course, they are a dating service!)

And how are you feeling today? Exhausted, confused, ecstatic, angry, ashamed... maybe all the same time, all at the same day. All of us at the group are there and feel like we don't identify ourselves as divorced. We write journals, one page for each topic. Courtship, years of marriage, breakup of marriage, mourning period, and regaining balance. I can see all five because my divorce is right there, page after page. But it seems like courtship was a day ago, and I have a pleasant smile remembering it. Her photos are on my entertainment shelf. It was special. She was so nice at 15 or 10 years ago, even five years ago! I remember the first time I saw her. Probably 1982 (so looo-ong!) I knew her. I thought that I understood her. Everything was nice! I photographed her with my Canon 35mm camera, and took a lot of pictures. She looked beautiful on the wedding. A photograph from years ago, I modeled her with a glass of red wine. It was my wife and the glass of wine – no scenes of flowers at a park, no mountains or a river beyond her, without friends or relatives. Just her... and a red wine glass. We had so fun! I (we) were truly in love. She later told me she was unhappy for 10 years or so of marriage.

The fourth chapter in the workshop reveals: Anger. The subject titled on the fifth chapter? More anger. I would add a sixth or seventh chapter: really, really more ANGER. "Anger is part of my life, Lord, I don't understand it and I don't like it, but it's there," says a poem, "Anger" by E. Witt. It was simple to how much I wrote, the number of expression points in my journal – three or four, to things like: She was so nice! She was kind, and she was so pretty. Add to chapter 5, "Regaining balance"... it was so clinical, so dry. No expression points. The sentences were shorter and briefer. "I can't regain a balance, although I can believe it now."

It's similar to aphasiacs with divorces. For divorces tell them, to favor "laugh a little – even at yourself. A sense of humor works wonders in many high-pressured situations." Divorce sounds like anger and aphasia versus stress. Woody Allen wrote, "Or than any other time in history, mankind faces a crossroads. One path leads to despair and utter hopelessness. The other, to total extinction. Let us pray we have the wisdom to choose correctly." My son Derek was 17, my daughter, Shannon, 14. My ex-wife didn't leave, at first only a mile away. My daughter and son were at the same house with me. But, "the love, affection and other emotional ties existing between the parties involved and the child," according to the state Friend of the Court. I thought about it. It was a dark and dismal house. They have to involve giving the love, affection and guidance, and continuation of the education and raising in the young children. Food, clothing and medical care for children must be realized. The moral fitness of the parties involved, plus mental and physical health of the parties, along with the home, school, and community record of the child. The court tells you: Don't pump the children for information about the other parent. Don't try to control the other parent through your children. Don't use the children to carry messages back and forth. DON'T ARGUE in front of the children! The court capitalized in their words.

Say good-bye. Before you can adjust your new family life, you must take to say good-bye, of the older life. This includes ridding yourself of feelings that keep you tied to the past. I know two men each divorced their own wives, each of them three years from then. When I talk to them, John and Frank, said their own ideas and their own ex-wives. Money, property, children had their ultimate ideas. After my divorce, money, property and children are not my ultimate ideas or my focal point.

Love

I don't what the odds are that a spouse divorced his/her marriage because of a stroke. But I bet it's a lot. I've had a stroke, and the spouse leaves. My divorce was midway. Divorce is to not accept the world. Feelings are neither good nor bad; they just *are*. You are not a "good" or "bad" person because you have these feelings. Marriage vs. divorce and love vs. hate are things that seem to be good/bad emotions. Married people have good and bad emotions.

Respect and accept each other in the group for what and who they are. Express your feelings, and don't be afraid to express bad feelings.
1) Recognize the feeling
2) Express the feeling
3) Clarify the feeling
4) Explain the feeling
5) Accept the feeling

Despite a divorce, or a job, say "I will take more risks. I will read the comics. I will find and eat at least five new health foods that I can actually enjoy. I will be thankful for at least three things a day. I will walk more places and take the stairs more often." And, lastly, "I will focus on what went right every day instead of what went wrong."

"There is no way to predict how you will
The reactions of grief are not like recipes,
with certain ingredients, and certain results.
Each person mourns in a different way...
You may be calm one moment – in turmoil the next.
Reactions are varied and contradictory
Grief is universal."
Living When, I Loved One Has Died by Earl Grollman

Our workshops or seminars are a way to ease our lives. It is what a person is reaching out, which they are a drowned man trying to grab a tossed lifesaver. It left me and so many others had to seek another chance. How could you describe your support group? An orchard maybe? Whenever I'm in this group I feel like a fragrant, healthy apple tree because of all the growing I've done and all the fruit I've been able to share. I think of seeing The Brady Bunch on t.v. I feel like I'm part of one big happy family. We're not perfect, but we love and accept each other. You get the message. Or you don't. A support group is not for you. Maybe you needed or wanted or just a conversation. Be a partner, not a therapist. Be a partner, not a date. Be willing to accept any form of communication, including writing or gestures. Make sure you sit down at least once a day and have a pleasant conversation. Or even an unpleasant conversation. Be willing to speak at a normal rate with normal pauses. Say, "How are you doing?" and believe it.

A really fast date

"QuickDate" or fastdater.com are dates from the Internet. An interested date would ask your email format. The format will include your hobbies, careers, food and cooking, restaurants, where you've lived, whether you travel, your personality and your hopes, and so on. But don't ask too much. You will talk for five minutes during the 10 women (or men) at a local restaurant or bar. Really, it's a "date" with five minutes or three minutes and the monitors can shush you after your time is longer than five minutes. If the five minutes went ok, you can email or phone again. At five minutes, you had to remember three things only: 1) first name 2) number (that's the way the monitors can help you) 3) what she/he wanted to say were interesting to you. Remember to jot down your paper if she was nice, if she was interesting, if she is pretty (be honest!) I was nervous! At first, I didn't try to talk with people. Five minutes was not too long, if you have aphasia. I told QuickDate monitors that I was tongue-tied, and told them that I had a stroke. They assured me it would be ok. They promised it would be fun, it would be better than I hated it. The dates won't hate you. People have dates blind or deaf during the QuickDates. In five minutes, I talked with my name and had two kids, I told them about my divorce, where I lived (in the neighborhood), the house, and hobbies, etc. Five minutes took a short time, and sometimes five minutes was long enough! An eternal was a long five minutes, not even talking with aphasia. Sometimes I told them that I had a stroke seven months ago. Don't talk about your stroke or, for example, your hospitalization or your disease or your heart attack, for your whole five minutes. I had aphasia, I said, in a few quick minutes. They don't want to hear all the details, even if it's meeting with my fellow stroke survivors. They really don't care. A stroke seemed the five minute conversation did not try to tell them the hospitalization – *who cares?* Instead you can talk about hobbies, sports, or your family or dream house, or your vacation. Five minutes were too long for talking a subject. Stroke is a burden. Five minutes was a downer, a bummer. The patients can detail their strokes at five minutes – how they stayed at the 10, 20 or 30 days in the hospital, how the operations were in the hospital, how their doctor is careful/happy/concerned. It's boring! Five minutes to talk about how you had an appendicitis operation or a hard labor with your pregnancy with your first child, or second child. Nobody cares. Enough is enough!

Medical evidence suggests a relationship from high levels of stress and increased risk for certain diseases. Sometimes involuntary impulses to organs in the body can increase blood pressure, heart rate, blood flow to the muscles, and breathing. Stress can be a survival mechanism. Chronic stress can create an adrenaline and cortisol, two hormones. They prepare to react, physically and emotionally. They can be manufactured high levels of stress. High blood pressure can also be from the heart, increases the risk for stroke by up to six times. This can lead to blood clots or hemorrhage. Know your triggers; stress can be a real and actual stroke.

Corticotropin and norepinephrine are hormones in the cortisol group. CRF is a highest suicide in depressive treaters. Depression is especially because of its known link with suicide. The comparison for these criteria is major depression. Show that while the symptoms are the same, the intensity and severity of major depression coupled with its chronicity distinguishes it from the reactive form. The prolonged duration of depression from a gradual onset reflects the patient's awareness. This interpretation supports a psychological basis for the depression of post-stroke. *It is not surprising to find depression in survivors of stroke.*

Stress for relieving

Stress-Relief, For Disasters Great and Small is about stress from a noted professional, Georgia Witkin, PhD, The Stress Program at Sinai School of Medicine, New York City. She wrote four of the reasons for stress:

Lack of control during or after the disaster. An accident or trauma threatens our control. We are drowning underwater. Events will have a more lasting negative effect that doesn't have control. For example, drivers or passengers in car accidents are eight times more likely to develop phobic travel anxiety than those who didn't have car accidents or plane casualties.

Persistent health problems before or after the disaster. Chronic pain disrupts sleeping, eating, sexual pleasure, concentration, and physical exercise. Is it any wonder that persistent health problems interfere with post-traumatic healing as well as everyday life?

Constant rethinking and rumination after the disaster. Negative interpretations can annoy memories (flashbacks). Strong predictors will increase the probability of someone suffering anxiety or post-traumatic stress disorder four to seven times until the first year. It may be that some victims over-generalize the danger that follows their disaster. It may be that seeing the fallout to be life-threatening when it isn't, or more frightening than it should be.

Financial loss or legal difficulties during or after the disaster. When we're "hit in the pocketbook", the economic bruises can last longer than physical bruises. We may feel we did not "take care of business", anticipate the disaster and protect our assets. If our self-worth is tied up in our financial success, there may be more guilt, anxiety, and depression after one year or longer. If financial trouble or litigation continues, the continuing reminded of the catastrophe will most likely interfere with a natural tendency toward symptom resolution.

His or her problem? It may be "fixed" or not. The problem is, that knowledge is power. Stress and depression make partners in a stroke. "We are built for disaster," wrote Witkin. My own stroke was a prescription for others that are disasters great and small: divorce, aphasia, stroke, mortgage, children (teenagers!), ex-wife, girlfriend, job and career, health insurance, money (always money!), problems with car and computer, etc. All Americans are faced with multiple reasons for anxiety. During these days, the escalating war in Iraq, pictures of American prisoners of war, a teetering economy, higher gas prices, the long-term threat of terrorist attacks at home and when traveling. It's already a pending disaster for us. But not all Americans are equally anxious. Not all fears scare the same events.
Whether you're lying wake nights with sweaty hands or headaches or you can coping calmly while the tumult may depend in

part on personality type. People react to stress and anxiety differently, depending in part on their personality style. John Oldham identifies basic personality styles in the New Personality Self-Portrait. He suggests a combination that might help one negotiate tough times, and what combination might be less helpful. Oldham is the executive director of the Institute of Psychiatry, Medical University of South Carolina, Charleston. Self-Portrait includes:

Conscientious. "The backbone of America," adults who tend toward hard work, who like order and detail and have strong moral principles and values.

Self-confident. Features self-esteem, this style welcomes attention and competition.

Vigilant. Independent, perceptive, loyal and cautious.

Sensitive. The "homebody," who builds a small world to call his own.

Mercurial. The "fire and ice" approach of one who lives life on a roller coaster.

Idiosyncratic. The "different drummer" who requires few close relationships and tunes in mostly to his own world.

People simply cope with threats differently. People might cope by trying to put a threat aside, ignoring it. They are the "repressors," while others are the "sensitizers". They highlight the danger in every little object. An USA TODAY/CNN/Gallup Poll shows that 75% of adults feel confident as a result of the 2003 war in Iraq, but 71% are sad, and 26% are afraid. The response that adults have to a long-term tension by their individual personality styles.

Those who study personality in all its complexity can provide guideposts to those who will do the best psychologically in the months, and possibly years, ahead. Researchers stress that personality involves much more than a list of traits or characteristics. Its genetic, environmental, hormonal, environmental, cultural and other ingredients that determine how an individual thinks, feels and behaves. Various tests, often with significant price tags. They are offered by different groups with different approaches to assessing personality types. Such tests might help you understand why you react to the world the way you do. Sources for additional information include the Internet, mental health counselors, the clergy, friends or relatives, human resources in your job, self-help videos and books. Many managers also make use of personality tests to help bring "harmony to the workplace." Harmony? That's a good one. Strangle your own employers? An adult's emotional stability determines how well he copes. But other personality factors will determine the form of happiness or anxiety.

One of the most noted personality assessments is the Myers Briggs Type Indicator (MBTI) from Consulting Psychologists Press. The MBTI develops 16 personality types from four building blocks, or ways of looking at the world, collecting and using information. Such a key can be helpful in understanding limitations that adults face in disturbing times, says Otto Kroeger, author of. *Type Talk at Work.* The MBTI is based in part on opposites such as "judgers" and "perceivers."

"Judging types prefer things closed and settled," Kroeger says. "Even if the news is bad, it gives them a sense of security." Their alter egos, the perceivers, are flexible. They go with the flow. "Sensors" would be less comfortable than "intuitives" with the ambiguities the country faces. Sensors like concrete information, while intuitives like imagination and possibilities. Stressors for me were jobs, divorce, doctors, bills, speech therapists, my two kids, my life love, physical health and mental health with or without aphasia.

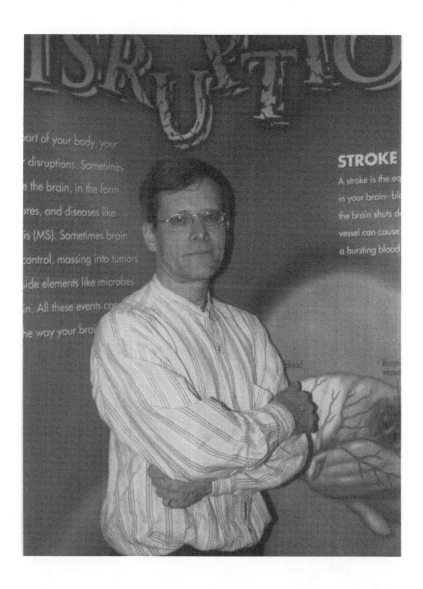

The author at a stroke exhibition at the Detroit Science Center.

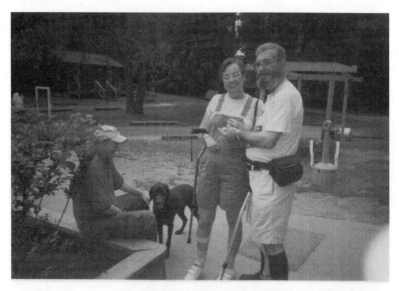

Jan and Phil at Camp Cavell.

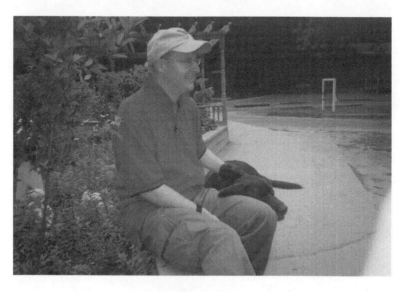

Jon at Camp Cavell.

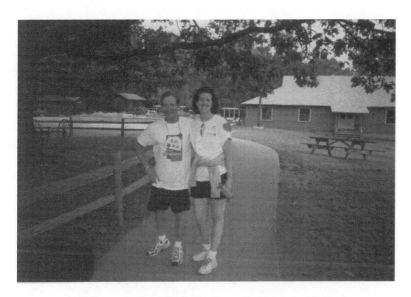

The author and a volunteer.

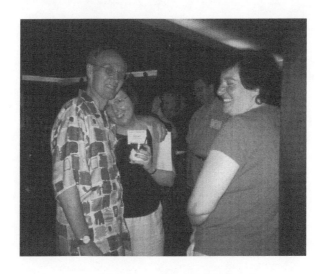

Mike and Sue McKesson
at the National Aphasia Meeting in Tampa, Florida.

Book Two

One year past – an overview

Chapter 1

Aphasia group activity

An aphasia group activity is a conversational focus for adult aphasic victors for using in practice groups. It requires little in the way of materials, although a blackboard is extremely useful so that participating members can follow along, visually as sentences are built. If desired, sentences can be recorded on paper for later practice or repetition. This is a sentence, beginning an exercise. The activity focus on building skills in the following areas:

Speech production
Sentence patterns
Question responses
Repetition
Word-finding
Conversational question-and-answer practice
Verb forms
Basic pronouns (you, we, I)
Basic locational prepositions (in, at)

Practice and drill are antidotes to the frustration of aphasia and apraxia. To start, choose a venue. Values can be any place you can think of, including countries, states, cities, towns, geographic locations, community locations (thinking of where; neighborhoods, blue collar, etc.) Where are you? What do you see? What do you see there, maybe in the supermarket, or at the zoo or the beach? That's not a question, but encourages one to build additional complexity into their sentences. I see lots of trees, grass and picnic benches, and bikes, runners, walkers on an asphalt path in the park. Further ways to increase difficulty and skill. Change verbs. Change questions. Add adjectives and switch them. There is no end to potential locations or venues.

Most people aren't familiar with aphasia. Most people have never heard of the word. The general public frequently misinterprets the difficulties an individual with aphasia is experiencing and may react as though the person is psychologically ill or mentally retarded. Feelings of social isolation with resulting emotional effects are common to individuals with aphasia. It means an individual has difficulty retrieving words for speech and usually has some problems understanding speech. The primary symptom is an inability to express oneself when speaking. In cases, reading and writing can be the more impaired language modality. In my three separate therapy classes, it's almost the same: repeating and redundancy. After my two years of my stroke, I am trying to pronounce sentences. I have to try talking. I'm lost with my friends. They can understand to me, but it's after communicating a few minutes or a few sentences. I want to talk, and they want to hear but they don't have the time. Communicating is talking, but can also be gesturing, body language, facial expressions, etc. You can gesture a middle finger extended. It does communicate, right?

A similar group lasts two hours each week. An aphasia meeting has about 12-15 persons, sometimes one or two speech therapists. A three-way group has from three to four persons with an activity. The one subgroup makes a sentence on a blackboard for verbs, nouns and propositions. A conversation with visitors depends on typically vacations or family. At another subgroup, people exercise "word power" according to Readers Digest monthly. All the visitors at the same meeting can join another subgroup. Every one has at his or her "two cents" for the limelight. Everyone have the chance, everyone gives an opportunity. Tell us: we can hear you. We want to hear from you. We will take a long time if you're slow or hesitant. My limelight was a risk for my chance at speaking for a aphasia meeting. It was too hard, too difficult at first. A member encouraged, "If you ever talk when you are thinking... it's a lot... you say what you like..." If I ever tell what my brain is thinking, it will be better for all of us. It almost has a brain with telephone lines, but only one that gives communication. They have a chance to hold the line. If it was too busy, hang up! All too much information gives them one, like a home with a single telephone line that is ready and willing to receive.

Support groups for aphasic meetings support these ground rules:

Let others share too. Each of you aware of allowing one another to have the necessary time to share.

Be on time to miss something (lunch maybe!) Two hours of a meeting was too long. I get away from it, getting a cup of coffee for an excuse.

Silence is ok, but everyone has a right to express him or her self. Or just remain silent. Respect this right for individuals can be quiet. Don't put them in the hot chair.

Express your feelings... but don't dwell on your hospitalization. It's hard to understand and tedious, too. Don't tell about every tiny incident. Forget it after you have told the same crowd.

Stick to the point, do not wander. Tell about your grand children, but not everyone, everything. Don't explain every person – if you have 13 or 15 grandchildren, their names, ages, sex, etc.

Share. Your experiences, feelings, and thoughts are open. You're on the stage. You're a chance for everybody that can hear it. "My name is... my stroke was..." (6 months or 6 years ago). We can hear it from your voice.

Chapter 2

Drugs for patients

"Pravachol" is one of a prescribed drug, it's not a nutraceutrical or a vitamin. It's needed if you don't have a less cholesterol and don't have it from diet and exercise. Pravachol (pravastatin sodium) in 40 mg tablets, made by Bristol-Myers Squibb Co. has been claimed to have be "the only cholesterol lowering drug proven to help protect against first and second heart attack and stroke." Pravachol (statin drugs as common as pravastatin) can cause liver problems. That's why users should have their blood checked from time to time to see if any liver damage is occurring. If it is, then stopping the drug stops the assault on the liver. From a rare side effect, these drugs can also damage muscles. An estimated 5% to 15% of patients report problems. They can be evidence that muscles are be detected with a blood test, discontinuing the drugs almost always ends muscle damage. Don't stop the drug without the doctor's approval. The drugs include Merck & Co.'s Zocor, Pfizer Inc.'s Lipitor and Bristol-Myers Squibb Co.'s Pravachol. An estimated 15 million Americans take cholesterol drugs, called statins. All statins reduce death from heart disease.

A jury cleared Bayer Corp. of liability in a 2003 $560-million lawsuit that accused the pharmaceutical giant of ignoring research linking the cholesterol-lowering drug Baycol to dozens of deaths. "The verdict validates Bayer's assertion that the company acted responsibly in the development, marketing and voluntary withdrawal of Baycol," the company said. The lawsuit was brought by Hollis Haltom, an 82-year-old engineer claimed that a muscle-wasting disease caused by Baycol severely weakened his legs. His lawyers had produced e-mails and internal documents to argue that Bayer didn't adequately warn doctors about the possible side effects of the drug before it was pulled off the market. Bayer was a Pittsburgh-based U.S. subsidiary of German pharmaceutical giant. Bayer AG had acknowledged the link between the drug and a side effect called rhabdomyolysis – a rare but life-threatening condition in which muscle cells are destroyed. In severe cases, the condition can lead to kidney failure. Baycol won FDA approval in 1997 and became the fastest-growing drug in Bayer's history. By the time it was pulled, it was Bayer's No. 3 seller, expected to earn $720 million that year with 6 million patients worldwide, including 700,000 in the United States. The pharmaceutical giant has paid $125 million to settle about 450 cases.

Centocor owned by Johnson & Johnson, developed ReoPro, a specific to a protein on the surface of platelets, which promote the formation of blood clots. By preventing platelets from sticking together, it reduces the chance of lethal cloth formation in patients undergoing angioplasty. Still other biotech companies are interested in cloning genes whose protein products are potential targets for new drugs, especially the genes for proteins usually found of cell surfaces that serves as receptors for neurotransmitters. Antibodies are molecules produced by the immune system. They'll bind to and identify invading organisms. Silver bullets they proved not to be, after decades of disappointment, they are just now coming to their own. It wasn't until 50 years ago, James Watson and Francis Crick wrote "Molecular Structure of Nucleic Acids" in issue of *Nature*. "We wish to suggest a structure for the salt of deoxyribose nucleic acid (DNA). This structure has novel features which are of considerable biological interest," they wrote. Fifty years ago, Watson said, "There remained, however, a single missing piece in the double helical jigsaw puzzle: our unzipping idea for DNA replication had yet to be experimentally verified." Nine years later, in 1963, Crick, Watson and Maurice Wilkins received their own Nobel Prize in Physiology or Medicine. "The discovery of the double helix sounded the death knell for vitalism." Said one American Center Society professor, "This is the story of DNA and therefore the story of life, sex, money, drugs, and still-to-be-revealed secrets. DNA is quite a molecule…" Money is lucrative or the Valhalla from all-things being biotech companies.

The cost of prescription medicines can quickly add up. Drugs can increase a high blood pressure, an anti-platelet and an anti-coagulant. Stroke victors with a second stroke have to take them for years. An Internet program makes it easier. The program, http/www.needymeds.com can be provided by a doctor and a social worker, gives them information and up to three months supplies: but only if you make a poverty wages and/or have a insurance that pays for your pharmacies. Some PAPs provide discounts on medication while others provide free medications to patients whom can't afford or who meet certain criteria. Each company had different rules. Qualifications are linked to your income level and insurance you receive. The web site offers free prescription drugs including http/www.phrma.org/pap (patient assistance programs). There are another couple of Internet web sites, http/www.rxassist.org/default.cfm and http/www.medicare.gov/prescription/home.asp. They don't offer drugs, they offer the contact for the pharmaceutical companies. The company Bristol-Myers manufactures Plavix (clopidogrel bisulfate) for stroke and heart disease patients. It's a blood thinner similar to fluvastatin, heparin and warfarin. While taking this medicine, if you have any kind of bleeding it may take longer than usual to stop, especially if you hurt yourself. Stay away from rough sports (fencing, not running) or other situations were you could be bruised, cut, or injured. I got bleeding (the first time) from shaving, but it wasn't seriously. A minor cut, at best. Side effects include: allergic reaction; blood in your urine; bloody or black, tarry spools; chest pain; fever, chills, sore throat; severe stomach pain; skin rash; and usual bleeding or bruising. I didn't have any side effects.

If you have problems with these side effects, talk with your doctor: diarrhea, indigestion, stomach pain; headache, dizziness; joint pain; or runny or stuffy nose, coughing. Aggrenox is a trade name with aspirin/dipyridamole (dye-peer-ID-a-mole) used to prevent strokes with blood flow disorders or a history of blood clots. You should not use this medicine if you ever had an unusual or allergic reaction to aspirin. Aspirin should not be given to children or teenagers with fever, chickenpox, or symptoms of the flu. Aspirin can cause stomach bleeding. Drinking alcohol can make this worse. If you have three or more drinks of alcohol every day, ask your doctor if you should take this medicine. Make sure your doctor knows if you are taking aspirin, blood thinners or arthritis (such as Motin, Anacin or Advil are trademarks.)

Experimental therapies based on a growing understanding of the brain. Bromocriptine (Parlodel) which is commonly used to help patients with Parkinson's disease is helping stroke patients with their speech pathology. The brain is thought to stimulate the drug dextroamphetamine, to get greater improvement in movement. The American Heart Association estimates that the cost of stroke-related medical care and disability, including lost productivity will be $51 billion this year. After aging the population the increasing incidence of declines in stroke rates. Seven hundred thousand Americans suffer strokes annually. 170,000 will die. Most private and government insurance programs provide for a wheelchair or cane, and leave patients to manage. The progress often stops at this time. Many experts predict that the best results will come from combining repetitive therapies with drugs. A sort of "cocktail" is with hard work and a dose of drugs.

Nutraceutricals vs. pharmaceuticals

There is a supplement food (not drugs) that attempts a limit to cholesterol. "Chlosterin" (trademark) is a non-pharmaceutic supplement. It produces Esterin in alcohol-based, purified water and alfalfa extract. "They hang their hats in chain pharmacies, strut their stuff in independent drugstores, and ply their trade in supermarkets and mass-merchandising outlets," said Allen Montgomery, founder and CEO of American Nutraceutical Association (ANA). "They can also be found in hospitals, academia, government, and home care organizations."

It advertises "removal of cholesterol from the body naturally." Cholesterin, as one, binds with cholesterol in the stomach unlike most other cholesterol supporting drugs. "Nutraceuticals" that supposedly work in the liver. It does not interfere with the metabolism of other drugs and nutraceuticals do not interfere with normal liver functions. It "neutralizes" cholesterol before it gets into your system, and reducing LDL by 21% while improving HDL by 26%. Cholesterin Plus is formulated to "healthy" people don't like the idea of ingesting medicines or don't have the money or drug insurance. An added benefit of non-flush Niacin (inositol hexanicotinate) will offer to managing cholesterol levels. They are for $30 for 60 tablets. That's a little higher than any prescription that Blue Cross insures it. The guidelines have a 36 million people with borderline high levels of cholesterol. The Cholesterin does not patients that have a high blood pressure, abdominal obesity, insulin resistance and smoking. Cholesterin Plus wants "to avoid prescription medications with harmful side effects." Without Blue Cross or similar health insurance, $30 is yet another expense. I am not a doctor, a medical researcher, nor a pharmacist. But I don't recommend it. It's manufactured from Vitamin Solutions. The statements were not evaluated by the Food and Drug Administration. They were not endorsed by JAMA but endorsed by JANA. The Journal of American Medicine Association, is the 1883-coveted publication. JANA is the Journal of American Nutraceuticals Association, which began in 1997.

People don't like taking drugs. Two headlines in the same daily newspaper: "Estrogen pills may hurt memory" and "Common asthma drug may boost the risk of deadly attacks or cardiac events." It's no wonder.

Research on many dietary supplements is contradictory. Even if some of the health benefits are true, it's difficult to determine the right dosage or to figure out the differences between brands on the market. Part of that problem may be solved for rules proposed by the Food and Drug Administration. The rules would set standards for making and labeling dietary supplements.

"Stroke" is not the word in the index from a book about the Atkins pro-protein, non-carbohydrate diet. It is healthy, or is it? I'm not a nutritionist. But an apple or a pear is ever harmful? Although popular diets like these leave many nutrition experts at a crossroads. Anything with white bread, waffles, cereal, and a bagel lists under the carbohydrates for almost dangerous identified by the Atkins diet. Trying a low-carb diet, as long as it was under their care and used to kick-start a more varied plan. Despite a flood of nutrition advice, people may actually understand very little about healthy eating. At least 87% eat healthy meals at least half the time. Fifty-two percent said they are eating in moderation.

"Cheerios" has 15% for fat from a 150 calorie serving (1 cup or 30 grams) with ½ cup skim milk. Total fat from Cheerios is 3%: saturated fat is 0%; cholesterol 0%, and 1% with the milk. The total carbohydrate is 10%. Ingredients include whole grain oats (including the oat bran). A breakfast with eggs and bacon, *everyday*, is good for you, according to the Atkins diet. I don't think so, even if you're losing weight. Protein is listed an excellent food. It's a diet intended to lose fat, therefore losing weight. But is it good for the heart, cholesterol, arteries, etc.? Atkins said it so. A million (or say) have tried his diet and said they lost weight. His book has been a best seller for years. Carbohydrates are the energy for runners. I believe that. People who eat so-called healthy diets but also are overweight probably are not active enough. Experts preach moderate food intake across the board, coupled with increased activity, even though both can be hard to achieve. Enriched breads, pastas, rice and cereals are good for aerobics, a system of physical conditioning involving exercises strenuously to increase respiration and heart rate; for example, swimming, running or calisthenics. Sticking with one serving of pasta will serve your carbo-load with your muscles. The same with sugar: meaning sugar, corn syrup, honey, high fructose, etc. From runners and just about who exercises, some sugar is allowed for healthy people (not diabetics). Persons have obesity, heart diseases and hyperactivity is not the problem with sugar. Eating sugar (and fat) were not eating well.

Herbal remedies have been widely used in foreign countries for years, and the products enjoyed a surge in popularity in the United States during the late 1990s. Sales of herbal supplements tallied $4.18 billion in 2001, up from $4.12 billion in 2000, according to the *Nutrition Business Journal*. But some studies have shown that the products aren't effective. Ephedra, promoted as a weight-loss aid, has been linked to health problems, including heart attacks and strokes and linked to deaths. "In general, the record clearly shows that herbal products are relatively safe," says Mark Blumenthal, founder of the American Botanical Council, a research and education group that supports responsible use of supplements. A lot of research has been done that has shown the herbs are effective for various conditions. But others say the answers on herbs don't compute. "It's clear they have some biological effect, but we really don't have a handle how significant that effect is," said David Schardt, senior nutritionist with the Center for Science in the Public Interest, a consumer group based in Washington, D.C. Many studies have raised questions about the effectiveness of herbs. In supermarkets, everything is "natural" or "organic" or "herbal" from parsley to steaks to shampoo.

Garlic can lower cholesterol. One government agency reviewed the literature and concluded that garlic may lower cholesterol levels in the short term, but there's no evidence that it lowers cholesterol in the long term. There are indications garlic may have other benefits health for your heart. How much garlic would be better? A couple of pills, or maybe a bottle of them or a couple of cloves?

Physician Tod Cooperman, president of http/www.consumerlab.com, knows how much the quality of products can vary. His company has tested more than 700 products since 1999. Many products failed to meet the standards the company established after reviewing the scientific data on the herb. Compared with vitamin and mineral supplements, herbals are the problems because of the complexity of manufacturing them. They need to have the right active ingredients that have been shown to be effective in clinical trials. Many of alternative medicines are low cost, non-invasive and non-toxics. Many offer alleviating chronic pain, dizziness and depression. A holistic healing center which allows conventional medical treatments or therapies, for complementary and alternative medicines (CAM). They can be:

- Alternative medical systems
- Energy therapies (herbs and supplements, or vitamins)
- Mind-body interventions (hypnosis)
- Biologically based therapies
- Manipulative and body-based methods (massage, acupuncture, chiropractic)

There was a notice in newspapers that chiropractors are harmful with stroke patients, mainly massaging within the neck arteries. The study found that stroke patients with torn arteries in the neck were six times more likely to have been to a chiropractor for an adjust in the preceding month. There can be an association between neck manipulation and strokes. Chiropractors can avoid neck manipulations. There may be imposters among the many honest and accredited practitioners. Imposters can prove and benefit their techniques and promise theirs a "cure" with its treatment that is only available in the yet another hospital in a foreign country. Don't spend your important health dollars for something that won't cure you.

Sham medications

High-priced prescription medications are proving irresistible to counterfeiters, who have sold fake, mislabeled and mishandled drugs. Many of the fakes are so good that pharmacists have trouble telling them from the real thing. Investigators and pharmacists say the problem of counterfeit or mislabeled drugs could spread beyond

the relatively few medications affected now unless state and federal regulators tighten requirements for the country's drug manufacturers. What some investigators are calling the biggest jump in bogus-drug cases in more than a decade, fueled by three things:
1. increasingly sophisticated forged labels
2. an abundance of small wholesalers buying and reselling medications
3. a growing number of expensive new treatments that can bring forgers large profits, with no concerns

The $192 billion worth of legal drugs sold in the United States annually, it's water under the bridge if you can think of counterfeit or adulterated drugs bought or purchased. The genetically engineered medications will hit the market in the coming years. Yet efforts to oversee the practice by requiring documentation every time drugs are bought or sold, all the way back to when they leave the factory. They've been fought by the wholesale industry, which states that rules are disturbing. The FDA has never fully implemented a 1988 law aimed at tracing drugs to their sources. The drug makers are not required to report cases to the FDA of counterfeit products for consumers.

Drugmakers and their wholesalers say they are doing everything they can to protect consumers. The American drug supply remains the safest "medicine cabinet" in the world. The solution they favor lies not in increased paperwork, but in better ways to mark drug packages so they can't be sold or faked. They also support efforts to make it more difficult to get a wholesaler's license. Most patients think prescriptions can be picked up at the drugstore directly from the manufacturer, at least half of the time.

The rest of the prescription drug market is more complex. Drugs go from manufacturers to smaller wholesalers, considered the secondary market, which then sell to pharmacies, clinics, and physicians. The secondary market is where investigators say most of the problems occur. Smaller wholesalers also sell to the major wholesalers, that buy a fraction of their drugs from the secondary market, newspapers reported on the drug market. Where medications may be more readily available or cheaper than buying directly from the manufacturer. Many secondary wholesalers are legitimate, operating clean warehouses with the proper temperature controls and computer systems to keep track of inventory. Statins improve mortality from heart attacks and stroke beyond what can be explained by the decreases they cause in cholesterol levels. The statins were increased 12.9% and increased $12.5 billion in overall drugs from 2001.

Chapter 3

Mechanical vs. drugs

A mechanical system is interesting can be searching and destroying thromboses or blood clots for patients having a stroke. The angioplasty is like a heart operation and a balloon. A procedure that cardiologists inflate the narrowed, clogged artery to clean out buildup and remove blood clots. "AngioJet" uses a suction saline fluid that is mechanically. The thousands of heart surgeons operate angioplasty but only a few dozens of neurologists have angiojet for strokes. This is a very small device that was approved in 1996 for using in blood clots, coronary arteries, balloon angioplasty (also with stenting), during heart attacks. More than seven million people suffer from coronary artery disease each year. This condition is caused by plaque buildup in the heart's arteries, and each year kills more than 500,000 Americans. Heart attack occurs when blood flow is blocked in a coronary artery. This most often occurs when a coronary plaque ruptures causing formation of a blood clot in the artery, slowing or completely stopping blood flow.

From the Minneapolis-based Possis Medical Inc., angiojet finds the Bernoulli effect produces inside an artery. The drug is to thin the blood during an operation, while the mechanical operation acts quickly. "Two passes of the 'AngioJet' catheter safely removed most of the clot and in approximately three minutes restored blood flow to the brain," Dr. Perl said. The patient was in very serious condition, unable to speak or move his body, and other slower therapies would have been much less effective and would have resulted in far more damage. "In 48 hours the patient was drinking on his own and talking with his family." The occurrence of thrombus during coronary interventions, especially patients with diffusely diseased "saphenous vein bypass grafts" associated with an increased incidence of procedural complications.

Bernoulli's law induces a vacuum with a steadily flowing fluid, performing a kinetic energy. The potential per unit volume is constantly at any point in the fluid (an 18th century Swiss mathematician/physicist Daniel Bernoulli). An aircraft wing's shape gives the lift. The Cleveland Clinic Foundation was the first successful use to halt an acute stroke involving the carotid system. The carotid arteries are the main vessels supplying blood to the brain. Clot formation in a carotid artery is often untreatable and can result in devastating physical and cognitive debilitation or death. The patient was as a result of showing signs of an oncoming stroke. A carotid artery was filled with a clot, which was triggering the stroke. Immediate removal of the clot by either surgery or drugs could not have been completed effectively in the time available to save the patient. Stroke treatment must be effective within hours. The angiojet has these parts:

Catheter – the thin, hollow tube that allows it to through an artery
Femoral artery – the patient's groin to be fed to the site of the blood clot.

Once activated, the pump set delivers a high-pressure saline solution through the catheter and out the saline jets into the artery. This creates a strong vacuum in the artery, which breaks up the blood clot and pulls it out of the body through the catheter and into the pump set.

Drive unit. This part of the angiojet powers the device and helps to assure the patient's safety.

The Bay Medical in San Francisco hospital used the first operation. Before placing a stent the cardiologist can quickly remove the blood, which will allow blood to flow freely again. Angiojet uses a very small catheter to navigate through the arteries to the area of blockage. When activated, high-speed saline jets create a localized low-pressure zone around the catheter tip. The difference between the low pressure at the catheter tip and the higher pressure in the artery will draw the clot into the catheter and out of the body. One of the benefits of angiojet is that it actually removes the clot from the body as opposed to just dissolving it and sending it downstream where pieces may cause additional blockages and complications.

"With angiojet we can remove a blockage of any size," says Bay Medical cardiologist James T. Cook, M.D. "Because clots are dissolved and vacuumed out of the artery, no blockage remains in the body." Angiojet has been shown to reduce the complications and severity of a heart attack and can decrease the length of stay in the hospital. Used before angioplasty, angiojet cleans out the blood clot in the blocked artery to minimize blockage of smaller arteries downstream by the breakup of the clot during angioplasty. Cardiologists at Bay Medical can also use angiojet and angioplasty to clean out blocked arteries and remove blood clots that certain medications for blood clots can't break up. "Angiojet removes much of the clotted, soft buildup in the arteries," says Frank Hedges, RTR, manager of Invasive and Non-Invasive Cardiology at Bay Medical. "Many times clots can cause buildup to return. Angiojet can clean out the artery and sometimes make the artery look brand new."

"Time is of the essence with heart attack patients," says Dr. Cook. "Initially angioplasty is the best way to evaluate and treat a person's heart, but angiojet may be necessary to completely clean out the arteries." While this procedure is excellent for many patients, it is not for everyone. Your cardiologist can determine which procedure is right for you.

Some of recent studies of certain patients who received a popular new drug-coated heart stent increased the last health warnings about the device. The Cypher stent is a tiny metal scaffold used for patients with heart disease. It opens a cleaned-out artery and, unlike other stents, emits a drug to reduce the artery will clog again. But that drug doesn't prevent a different risk posed by all stents. Blood clots that form around the device and can cause another heart attack. In more than 60 cases, the device was associated with the patient's death. Clots occurred up to 30 days after the stent was implanted.

Chapter 4

Computers and software

There is a way to speak better. Computer software is another way to abundant English as a second language in the bookstores, libraries, computer shops, etc. It costs $25-$30, sometimes even less. Often it is specifically to understand aphasia, but a lot of the software does not discern of aphasia as a handicap. As a second English language (individual CD language in Portuguese, French, German, Spanish, Russian, etc.) it does an aphasic patient, everyone learns how to speak English – whether their homes in New York (*New Yawk*). "Instant Immersion" is a Blackstone Multimedia Inc. and is four CD-ROMs with a brief (one page) hard printing. As an added bonus, it had an 8-in-1 English dictionary. It comes American English and British English. It lets you choose your native language to understand the starting directions and the meanings of English words. For example, there are categories from animals to vegetables, from sports to seasons (winter, summer, etc). The compartment subwords branched into recreation words: backpack, bowl, karate, relax, skateboard and volleyball. It's simple and easy. They have Windows 95/98/2000/NT, or the same programs with XP or ME. "Insert CD-ROM into your CD-ROM drive." I can do that. Left the mouse click RUN and run the speech exercise in E:/speech32/exe (on my computer it was a D:). The same software equals the study session on a non-PC: i.e. Apple MacIntosh.

On a restaurant, words are on the screen. Pictures are people eating their dinner. There are a window and plants and one along a wall. The question is "are windows in the walls at the restaurant?" Do plants growing around the interior? A sign said "No smoking." Do the customers are smoking their cigarettes? Cars have a whole language. The car engine, cylinders, transmission, shifter, windshield, gear shifter, gas pedal, power brakes, etc. For the British English, they don't have a hood on top of the engine as does American English – they have a bonnet. In American English, it's a windshield, not the front window or glass in the car. The windshield wipers do not have a "glass cleaners" There is a word, another better one. You tell them you need new glass cleaners and won't know. They can understand it, maybe. But it gives under American English as "tyres" as "pneumatic, round rubber." A mistake in their language: tires vs. tyres. The best part of this software is the Speech Solution, which is a treasury for them with aphasia. Sample words (video and audio) gives *under, suggestion, trouble, blunder and construction,* etc. "Comparative word" practices words with similar sounds. Under "Sentences" practice sounds used in sentences; i.e. Paul got his car with his father. The small dog loved to walk in the fall leaves in the park. Paula's small daughter caught the ball for the first time. Sounds "Speech Solutions" give it a sound or ability with lips and tongue. "Comparative" just as it sounds: dog/dug; balk/buck; hot/hut; sawn/sun.

Listening discrimination improve your listening comprehension. I am sure that you cut/caught the bread. The lunch/launch was very tasteful. The dog took his ball/bowl in the backyard. The cost is $29.99, a steal for this 4 CDs. It is available from the public libraries. English is a second language, for me. You can try it in the library, before you can buy the software. Aphasia is a very thin niche, and public libraries generally do not have books or software for them. Second language in English is out there for books and software, probably in the Bargains or the Price Busters bin at Comp USA or sold supplements with software. You can understand English as your "second" language.

TriplePlayPlus! is a Random House/Syracuse Language Systems Program for Windows 95/3.1 a CD, a microphone, user's or technical manual for $79.95. It also has "SoundStart," the key sounds of English, a speech recognition, it rewards your correct pronunciation, and record/playbook that compares you to a native speaker, in adult male, female or childish). The Syracuse Program incorporates a single CD-ROM and a 70-page user's manual, it costs around $15. Use the SoundStart to improve 50 common words in English and to practice automatic speech recognition and record-playback. The CD gives you feedback on your pronunciation. Use record-playback to compare or contrast your voice. Choose your voice classification, if necessary, by clicking on either a child, female or male. Check the onscreen microphone on/off control, which is located on the bottom right corner of your screen. The small arrow should be pointing at the green light, indicating that the control is turned on. If you see a large arrow pointing to the microphone icon, it means that this feature is turned off. Click on the microphone icon, the large arrow will disappear and the small arrow will point to the green light, or On the position. It seems like hard, but it's easier and can be fun. Can it be better for relearning your English? It takes you originally several years, don't expect to have one or two lessons. Keep learning!

A microphone comes with many personal computers, or you can buy it from $10 to $30 at computers stores or Radio Shack. Of course, you will need speakers. If they are not with your computer, you can buy options. They can be $30-$50 for speakers, ready at computers or electronics stores. To understand in the letters and sounds, click on any word to hear it pronounced. Click on "see clue" in the picture window on the right side of the screen to see a picture of the word. Click on the arrow to the right of the word several times. Each time you click, you will hear an additional word that uses with the corresponding letter. Click on the letter key to the left of a word. An example will open it showing of the various sounds that can be represented by the letter. Click on any item, to see other examples that show the same agreement of the letter to the sound. Click on any of these examples to hear how the word is pronounced. Click on *go*. The game screen (or picture window) will display a set of words.

You will hear a word. Click on the word that matches what you just heard. If you are correct, the window will open and show a picture of the item or object. If a word is repeated, click on "hear." The game or puzzle continues until you have found all the words.

You will hear two or three clues describing a geographic location on the map. An extra clue is also available. Click on the blue pin in the appropriate location. If you are not correct, try again. The game continues until the pins have been changed from blue to red. Bungalow Software bundles software for speech and language. Designed and tested by speech therapists, it is in use for therapy at home or independent practice. It has computer-based activities for word retrieval, articulation, reading and auditory comprehension, memory, aphasia and apraxia, logic and reasoning, cognitive deficits, and voice disorders. Terri Nichols worked as a speech language pathologist, husband and partner Clay, an engineer who created some programs for Terri's patients. "Patients rarely get as much speech therapy as they'd like," said Nichols. "But it can help even more during therapy… it can't replace a therapist, but it's excellent for the intensive practice that speech therapy requires."

Speech therapy with therapists is a lot of money, relatively, even after paying 80% of health insurance. Computer requirements any Windows PC, with CD-ROM and sound card (Microsoft Windows 95, 98, ME, 2000 or XP). Hard drive is a 10 Mb of free space per program and 32 Mb RAM, with a 166 Mhz or faster Pentium 1.

It was helping patients to use the computer. But some patients have difficulty with the computer. I know. They might be confused by looking up at the screen, then down at the keyboard. Sometimes an arm or hand doesn't have movements among stroke survivors. They might have difficulty with the mouse or keyboard. I used a computer almost for every day, 20 years or more, but I have some trouble with some programs or files, either introductory English as a second language or aphasia. Recommended is:

Use a "touch screen." Caregivers should stand behind or to the side of the patient, with your hand occasionally on their hand atop the mouse.

As they move their finger or hand near the screen, you move the mouse pointer. Tell them the pointer will follow their finger. Have fun with it. Take a game or think about another game or word puzzle.

When they touch the screen, you move the mouse to click on what they touched. They only need to look at the screen.

Once they're comfortable with that, gradually have started to use the mouse or keyboard. Show them how moving the mouse moves the cursor on the screen.

If they get confused, go back to start, or take an hour break or lunch break.

A touchball can be better for some than a mouse. Moving a mouse uses your hand although a trackball solves all of this: use of one finger from the ball to a button to click. They can be bought from $30 to $60 at a computer store. Terri Nichols, MS, CCC-SLP, summed the benefits of technology, in conversations for annual speech and language conferences. They are including:

a.   Builds self-esteem
    i.   Allows independent practice with objective feedback
    ii.   Conserves health insurance benefits
    iii.   Allows unlimited drill on specific levels
    iv.   Simultaneous multi-sensory input
    v.   Compensates for physical deficits
    vi.   Technology use can be an excellent functional goal in itself

A "barrier to technology" expect aphasia patients leading them fear and intimidation, the limited access or space, physical limitations and the past experience of "bad" technology. Computers can be intimidating to anyone, even if you haven't had a stroke or brain injury. Here are the following computer tips:

Mark important keys on the keyboard (such as the space bar and enter key) with colored tape, to make them easy to spot. If you don't have colored tape handy, a few magic markers and some masking tape will do. If necessary, buy large-type keyboard stickers (ZoomCaps are $14.95 for upper case and $19.95 for lower case, either white on black or black on beige).

Introduce the task as if it were a pencil and paper task first, pointing to items on the screen, and encouraging the client to point to the screen as well. Be sure they grasp the language aspect of the task before you teach the computer aspect of the task.

Demonstrate the computer task several times.

Provide hand-over-hand assistance for the first few items.

Step back and provide supportive encouragement while you let the client try a few on their own.

If the client gets a wrong answer, positively reinforce that they are using the computer correctly.

Set the task options for a difficulty level which results in 65-90% accuracy.

With the software bought from stores or from web sites, pathology-driven software cost is better and almost available and affordable. Among the case in this patient, a 39- year-old male, had severe aphasia crossing all modalities. He had no motoric deficits from the CVA, observed his therapist, so was discharged directly from acute care to home with his parents. Before he had his stroke, he was a computer programmer. His initial evaluated data:

Auditory comprehension
Single word comprehension/picture identification: 75%
Yes/No questions: 65%
1-step instructions: 0%
Verbal expression:
Spontaneous naming: 0%
Sentence completion: 0%
Word repetition: 90%
Reading comprehension:
Picture-word matching: 96%
Sentence comprehension: 70%
Written language:
Single word naming: 0%
Copying: 100%
Signature: functional

The outpatient treatment began at a frequency of twice per week, for 1-hour sessions. Because the patient was computer literate, and was still able to install software and use familiar Windows-based programs. The patient independently targeted reading and writing skills at home. He used Aphasia Tutor 1 and Aphasia Tutor 2 from Bungalow software. The patient brought printouts of his performance data to each treatment session. They were used to determine when he should progress to the next level. He was encouraged to proceed quickly, said the therapist, to the fill-in levels, and resort to multiple choice only after two failed attempts from typing the words. During a re-evaluation, after 20 treatment sessions and two months of home computer practice with aphasia software, the patient indicated with gestures and verbalization that it was not noticed that writing words he had practiced on the computer.

Auditory Comprehension Initial Progress
Single word comprehension: 75% 100%
Yes/No questions: 65% 80%
1-step instructions: 0% 90%

Verbal expression:
Spontaneous naming: 0% 40%
Sentence completion: 0% 70%
Word repetition: 90% 90%

Reading comprehension:
Picture-word matching: 96% 100%
Sentence comprehension: 70% 100%
Written language: Initial Progress
Single words: nouns: 0% 40% 100%
Single words: verbs 0% 25% 80%
Written sentence completion: 0% 20% 100%

"The Written Language testing was done with pencil and paper, rather than typing on the computer," Nichols said. "The patient continued to receive therapy services for 15 months, at decreasing frequency, for a total of 54 visits. He currently converses primarily in single words and phrases, and occasional sentences. He is reading novels, and has learned a new programming language. He was re-hired by his former employer as a contract programmer for 3 months, and vocational rehabilitation paid for a consultation visit to his employer for recommendations to maximize communication."

The therapy category has an articulation (apraxia, dysarthia, etc.), word retrieval (expressive aphasia), reading comprehension (receptive aphasia), and so on. Voice therapy gives the pitch, loudness and tone of the voice. Software is controllable by the survivor so it is highly flexible and eliminates peer pressure and the fear of failure. Adults accept it more easily than workbooks. Some students feel the workbooks are "child's play." Variable programs provide different training. Someone with aphasia might use a series of programs designed to increase first their skills in letters and words. The newest software uses digitized speech to reproduce a human voice, then plays back the stroke victor's spoken response for comparison. Change difficulty by presenting any or all of these cues: written word, spoken word and pictures. Speech clarity or articulation give the student's lessons for consonant-vowel syllables. In the middle, words organized by beginning sounds (sh in shut or shim), and words organized by ending sounds (sh in wish and rush).

Lessons for speech clarity and word retrieval including pictures and words of nouns, pictures and words for action verbs, and words for abstract concepts (still harder for me after two years). Speech pathologist William Pitts, MA, CCC, SLP designed another aphasia software over a ten year period in association with the Easter Seal Society of Greater Cleveland.

Parrot is aphasia software, too. Parrot Software has launched a web site featuring 60 different software programs for the remediation of speech, cognitive, language, attention, and memory deficits seen in individuals who have suffered aphasia from stroke or head/brain injury. The treatment path, researchers agree, for individuals with head injury and stroke is usually a long one requiring many hours of rehabilitation. That means a lot of time and a lot of money. Recommended for letter and word recognition, word retrieval, typing, written naming, reading words, and grammar. This Out Loud version has everything in the regular version plus it speaks the cues and answers. It runs $149.50 for the home version (in 2003), with $169.50 for the deluxe version, and $199.50 for the "pro" version. That is cheaper for one speech therapy. There is also aphasia tutor, word retrieval (recall), spelling (my favorite, I was a champion in the sixth grade spelling bee!) and reading-pronouncing words. A sentence system and functional reading, story reading, vocabulary and understanding questions, along with categories, traffic signs and direction or instructions with a manual or in a recipe. Another was memory, reasoning and reading comprehension, more thorough complex books.

Cost prohibits survivors from seeing specialists for more than 2-3 times a week. Medical insurers including Medicare have significantly limited reimbursements for long-term care. The Parrot Software Internet site is a relative, extended-care option. Customers subscribe to on-line service for $24.95 per month (2003 prices) with the first week free as a trial. Performance is recorded for each user in the form of a web page that can be accessed by the user or the clinician. My classes at Wayne State University used the Parrot Software. It was fun and was challenging. We also had a therapy or a combined class time with several students and two or three clinicians. It also gives a touch screen for $335 (15-inch) to $535 (21-inch) but can also be at a computer- or office supplies store. If you're older (age 50 or more) you'll want the bigger screen. My old Packard Bell monitor, 15 years old, is merely 12-inches. Try to read the newspaper on its monitor – the words are tiny. Both my eyes are adequate. Thank God for my eyesight, knock on wood.

Individual classes are at least $99 apiece. Premium software packages is priced at $6,000 for a set of 80 individual programs. The "deluxe" software package is $2,500, 40 programs. The programs available on this web site mirror activities of speech-language pathologists, occupational therapists and neuro-psychologists. Programs were designed for the non-computer user and free technical support is available via a toll free number and soon through a sort of "Netmeeting." There are lessons of many difficulty levels and programs report performance at the completion of each lesson. Parrot Software has been developing treatment software for people with communication problems since 1981. These programs have been purchased by almost every medical care facility in the U.S. and in many English, French, Spanish, Russian, Portuguese and Danish speaking countries. Parrot Software provides this Internet as an alternative to purchasing software. The software provides products for patients with head-injury and stroke. For additional information, complete descriptions of the products they offer are at its web site, http:/www.parrot-software.com. You can request a free CD-ROM to install the Internet Subscription Service by calling 1-800-PARROT-1 (1-800-727-7681).

Example of logical thinking: Users are asked to move a picture to a certain location. Lesson types include: Put baseball on a red square that is not even numbered; Put baseball on a red, even numbered square; If 10 is an odd number then put baseball below box 10.

Otherwise put baseball above box 10; if box 18 is blue or box 4 is green then put baseball in the upper-right hand corner. Otherwise put baseball in box 4. If box 19 is yellow put the baseball in the upper right hand corner. Put a baseball in box 19. If box 19 is not yellow put baseball in the upper right hand corner. Otherwise, put baseball in box 19. Cumulative progress reports can be printed. Minimum requirements are Windows 98 or higher, a Pentium II processor at 233MHz, 128 megabytes (MB) and 64 MB RAM. A microphone with a high quality device with built-in noise filters is also recommended.

Examples: making change for spending money, picture identification, sequence of events (mail a letter, put letter in envelope, write letter, etc.), logical thinking, cause and effect (your bed pillowcase cover will fade, the pillowcase will shrink, etc.), spelling and word finding, reading comprehension, sentence completion, word order, cooking time management, traffic signs, math story problems using a calculator, multiple meaning words, antonyms and synonyms, etc. It's time for realizing your life. A mistake I noticed under Presidents placed Richard Nixon to precede John Kennedy. Misspelled tennis Wimbledon in absence of "Wimbleton." British, especially tennis fans, shouldn't misspell Wimbledon, . Mr. Stallione the actor is mistaken: remember Sylvester or Sly *Stallone.* "Seperate" was originally misspelled for separate. There are many typos of this software, so beware from the software manufacturers. The test and records a percent at your own initiative.

An unlimited, independent therapy program is used for program specially-designed by speech therapists. There are home and professional versions. There are easy to use for speech, word retrieval, aphasia and apraxia, reading and memory, to learn at the leisure of one's home. It's not say whether Mac or IBM-clones, or what Microsoft versions are on. The URL address is: http:/ www.strokesoftware.com.

The "old fashioned" VCR tapes are very inexpensive, and easily located. Basic English, English as a Second Language is in all three units: basic, intermediate and advanced. For English, it's a problem with me. I could be saying French or Spanish or German. But the problem with VCR tapes is that they are boring. With a remote control, you can stop it and rewind it, in case you missed it or didn't get it. Quicker than VCR tapes, are DVDs or CD-ROMs. You'll have to be really good with your hands if you want to replay tapes, and be part of their dull and old-fashioned 1989-era. Letting it go you get the chance of missing an integral part of the tape. "All grammar structures are clearly illustrated with colorful video graphics," describes the packaging of this VCR tape. Really? Perhaps in the 1990-style. "Detailed explanations are given, and demonstrated on the chalkboard." Literally, they are demonstrated on a chalkboard – you can almost see students yawning in the school classrooms. You can see videocassettes at a local public library. Newer versions can be available with software stores. If you want a video or VCR tape, they are available and relatively inexpensive. I couldn't run it more than once, it was so terribly tedious. For exercising, there are plenty of VHS from Kathy Ireland to Richard Simmons and Denise Austin. Hear them or have them on your daily exercise in morning or after dinner.

Non-fiction and fiction books for CDs and audiocassettes give a reward, especially for aphasia patients. Actors-actresses and authors give the dramatic reading for everything from Star Trek episodes to John Grisham and Ken Follett bestsellers to William Shakespeare and the Bible. It makes happy to people who cannot visually or read hundreds of pages in the books. There are hundreds or even thousands at the bookstores or libraries. Dr. Wayne Dyer and Dr. Susan Jeffers, are two of many writers that give them helpful suggestions and information. They can be heard in the car audio or personal cassette and/or CD player. You can take them with you, to be exercised and running, bicycling, during the cleaning your garage or home, grocery shopping, gardening, in the sunny day around your swimming pool, or while you are relaxing from a busy day, from an hour or two before sleeping. Once you have read best-selling author Dr. Dyer, you can understand these life-changing secrets:

- Choose, control and direct your destiny
- Manage your emotions
- Have faith and follow your dreams, regardless of outside influences or circumstances

You will understand "…where you will discover why neuroses and anxieties service a purpose there – and why they do not on Earth," said Dr. Dyer… "who reveals some all-important secrets to enjoying every moment of every day."

Dr. Jeffers said, "It's now time to begin flexing the muscles that lifts you to the best of who you are. I invite you to push through your fear and find that place of strength that lies within you… the place where you can find all the confidence and love that you will ever need as you walk through the journey of life."

From $10 to $20 you can buy, or buy gifts for audiocassettes for his or her birthday and Christmas, or your friends and relatives. I can't exercise or run listening to books on tape. It's better with a quiet environment. I like hearing music with running. I listen to rock 'n roll. I recommend my favorites: the Doors, Pat Benatar, the Rolling Stones, Santana, Jimi Hendrix, Bruce Springsteen, Tom Petty, Hank Williams Jr. or Kid Rock. Dyer is slow (compared to Springsteen!), harder to understand and even difficult, for me, if you can't see his gestures or facial results and his fingers and hands. When I was walking around the neighborhood or along to the park or beach, he (and all authors) will be easier to understand his books. You can run an audiocassette, twice and more, to "read" his tape. You can rerun a tape but it's harder and more boring to reread a page, or reread a book. Jeffers' gentle voice is reading on her videocassette. Soothing music and her pleasant words are not the same when you're running miles and miles and need Z.Z. Top! Give them a try, and you will probably have a niche for exercise or relaxing, on the sofa or on the recliner.

I am a single reader. Before reading a book, for example, I shut off the t.v. or the radio. I have to concentrate my few neurons. It distracts reading a newspaper or book. I have to at least lower the volume.

Before, I could read and watch t.v. or listen to the radio. I have too few neurons in my brain, I think.

Because from the aphasia programs vary so widely, not all of these products are appropriate for every person with aphasia, said Mary Boyle, a member of American Speech-Language-Hearing Association. It's best to get recommendations from your speech-language pathologist before investing money in these products you can help them or take them back. Similarly to software or books, CD-ROMS and videos, the problem is looking for aphasia. Looking "aphasia" subjects at a library or bookstore, where do you find them? Where do they store them? Under arts/literature in a category? Technical/science? Or medicine? In a subgroup, or within a smaller subgroup like "stroke"? They can be found in niches, but where? In occasional, you can find them under the topic "medicine." Or, perhaps, in English or in a language. There aren't a lot of them, just a few in bookshelves of categories and subcategories.

Chapter 5

Running away from stress

"Running! If there's any activity happier, more exhilarating, more nourishing to the imagination, I can't think of what it might be... The structural problems I set for myself in writing, in a long, snarled, frustrating, and sometimes despairing morning of work, for instance, I can usually unsnarl by running in the afternoon."
Joyce Carol Oates
Writer magazine

Why does running is like writing? My two careers resemble one another. I wrote stories at the age of 12 but started as a career at age 20. Almost when I ran (I was not a jogger; *Runner's World* is the national magazine, not Jogger's World). They are like hobbies, but it's a lot more. I got the same interests around 1974, with both writing and running. I can remember the first run, at a park on an asphalt path. It was warm, a summer day. I wore blue jeans, not even wearing shorts! I didn't own running shoes. I did maybe running a quarter mile. But I tried it, a second time, and a third. Almost after 30 years, I am still running. Sons and daughters, teachers or engineers, wives and husbands, RUNNERS... that's an ad from Runner's World: "It's what we love that defines us." Physical inactivity is one of the major risk factors for heart disease and stroke. I didn't run marathons (26.2 miles) at first, didn't even run a half-marathon (13.1 miles) 10 years after running. I ran as much as the Bobby Crim Festival 10 miles annual road race in Flint, Mich., since I was a "serious" runner. The race course has 10 miles, 10K, 1 mile, and a race named for teddy bears under-10 age for kids. That's 10 miles was the Crim was long enough! At running 10 years, 10 miles, that was I had finished. I still kept 10K runs, 6.2 miles, and the "little" Dodge Park (Sterling Heights, Mich.) race in my neighborhood in June, at just 3.1 miles, for at least running 15 years. It was fun! I didn't care, didn't have a person I was taking a chance, or trying him to "win" in the race. If you are in a field of 10,000 (the national Crim race) or 100 runners (Dodge Park), the contest is the same. You find a race against time. You find it's better than last year. You finished and that's ok. "How did you do?" you asked runners. You don't ask: Were you first? (or the 10th, or the 100th?) "I finished," you said. "That's enough!" Now, it's a half-marathon: 13.1 miles. Next was a marathon in Cleveland, only 180 miles from my house in Michigan, in April 2004. There were plenty of runners who drove or flew a plane for marathons. In 2002, there were more than 31,000 finishers in New York City's marathon. There were at almost in Chicago. Detroit's marathon was almost 3,000 runners, 26th in the United States. I'm thinking... and I'm still running. Dr. George Sheehan told his last column on running, before he died in 1993, "There can be no let up. If I do not run, I will eventually lose all I have gained – and my future with it... An achievement, no matter how magnificent, will eventually decay if not preserved by constant care."

Some hints are good, some are not good. Keep hydrated. Drink a glass of water a few minutes before you start, carry a minute before you start, carry a bottle or, if you can, stop at fountains on the way. It's a good idea. Don't drink constantly, just keep hydrated. Walk in well-traveled areas during daylight hours. Well, there are the paths are untraveled. During a time of the evening, or at the night is your only time. During the winter, in Chicago or Detroit or New York, it's dark by past 5:30 p.m. When are you supposed to run? I've run at many areas, and all times: morning or evenings. Walking is a relatively ease alternative to plopping down in front of the television. But running is a better choice. People (even doctors) can say that running is a bad effect. It strains the feet, hamstrings, thighs and knees of a runner, they can say. Balderdash (and other synonyms!) I've been running for 25 years and more, on concrete streets or a sidewalk, not just grass. Don't struggle yourself. Don't try to perspire. Oh, please! Sweat, if it's okay for you. You'll have to learn running. It's easier for you. Some doctors – most – don't exercise and don't run. Listen to other runners. Doctors who run and write are only a few mortals!

Among the running shoes is Nike, Asics, Adidas, New Balance, Saucony, Reebok, Brooks... they are all good shoes. I tend to like Nikes and Sauconys, but I am not a bit fussy. I'm not an exercise instructor or personal trainer, I was a runner 30 years plus. Any on the "clearance shelves" at a sporting goods are quality and worthy shoes, for around $50 – unless you have especially bad feet or you buy shoes an odd size. You don't have to pay $100, unless you really want to and you can afford it. Like automobiles, they make new models every year or two years. How to buy comfortable shoes is simple:

Have your feet measured while you're standing

Rely on fit, not size

Wear both shoes in the store and walk around

If your feet are different size, buy the pair that feels best on your larger foot

Don't buy shoes thinking you must break in – shoes should be comfortable immediately

Shop shoes late in the day; feet often swell by late afternoon or after work (morning in case your job shifts are in midnights)

Buy shoes that don't pinch your toes (women: they're *not* high heels)

Try on shoes while wearing the same type of socks you'll normally wear with them

Don't forget the usual tips:

Warm up. Stretch a half-mile into your walk and again when you're done, for greater flexibility. Stretch your calves, hamstrings, hips and thighs.

Keep hydrated. Drink a glass of water a few minutes before you start, carry a bottle or, if you can, stop at fountains on the way.

Don't overstride. It jolts your joints and slows you down.
Don't use ankle or hand weights. They interrupt the natural flow
of your walk.
Some people wear sweatshirts and pants for running: you *don't*
want to perspire or lose your own moisture.

Stress occurs when the body responds to a physical, chemical
emotional or environmental stimulus. Increased stress activates the
area of the brain that sends involuntary impulses to organs
throughout the body – higher blood pressure, heart rate, breathing,
metabolism and blood flow to the muscles. Depression more than
triples the likelihood of dying in the 10 years after a stroke, and
treatment with antidepressants may improve survival. The link
between depression and fatal heart attacks is well known. As stroke
research catches up, it's showing that depression also can be lethal
for adults who suffer strokes, says Robert Robinson, chairman of the
University of Iowa Medical School's psychiatry department. He
spoke at the American Psychiatric Association meeting in San
Francisco. About 20% of adults develop major depression after a
stroke. "We know from family members that the vast majority never
had a depression before," says Robinson. Depression is cited in cases
of 70% to 80% stroke patients. In 2000, 700,000 Americans suffered
strokes; 167,661 died.

If brain imaging within two months, shows the stroke occurred in
the left frontal cortex or the basal ganglia of the left hemisphere,
patients are at high risk for depression. About 70% will become
depressed, compared with 10% of those with damage to other areas
of the brain. Particularly vulnerable to depression are those who
already had tissue shrinkage in the left brain, often caused by a birth
injury or air pollutants.

A study of 100 stroke patients followed for 10 years, depressed
adults were 3½ times more likely than the non-depressed to die, even
after accounting for other key influences on health. In a field of 103
patients, depression for cases can prompt weight gain, make blood
"stickier" so it clots more easily and stubbornly, and trigger the

release of inflammatory molecules that clog arteries — all potential risk factors for stroke. Research suggests that depression make persons more vulnerable to strokes.

Adults can pay a high price for not dealing with such chronic distress. Long-term stress releases brain chemicals that can be toxic, contributing to everything from headaches to heart attacks, says Paul Rosch, clinical professor of medicine and psychiatry at New York Medical College and president of the American Institute of Stress. The Institute's Web site, www.stress.org, lists such conditions. About 60% of visits to health care professionals are "in the stress-related, mind-body realm," worsening problems from sexual performance to insomnia, says Herbert Benson, president of the Mind/Body Medical Institute and co-author of *The Break-Out Principle*. The first problem for researchers seems elementary: agreeing on a definition. "Stress is different for each one of us," Rosch says. Giving a speech can be terrifying for some, but a delight for those who love being the center of attention.

Researchers don't talk about eliminating stress. Stress is an unavoidable consequence of life, of the human condition. It is a virtuous action, sparking necessary to react to danger or improving — to a point — performance and productivity. Sometimes an employee actually wants to perform and can produce because of deadlines.

But chronic stress can leach the joy from daily living. Researchers are finding new clues, knowing how to handle it, and preventing it is proving to be significant. The core cause of much stress is the sense one is not in the driver's seat. Literally, a not old woman, age 40, was in her driver's seat with a new road test. She had to apply a driving license. She was nervous, and she was angry with her pending failure. All the clinical and lab research shows that the perception of not having control is very stressful. The way to turn a stressful incident into something that is not stressful is to regain a sense of control over it. While you may not control events (road test and driving license), experts say you can control your reactions (your driving).

Our new understanding of fear and phobia also led to pharmaceutical for post-traumatic stress disorder. Beta-blockers can suffer traumatic events; that emotional excitement triggers the memory-enhancing cycle all over again, making the traumatic memory even stronger. By preventing the reaction, beta-blockers keep the memory from forming deeper grooves in the brain, like skid marks or a scratch in an audio record, making post traumatic stress symptoms less severe. Our great elegance is in the way this system has evolved, with its complex of instinct and learning. We can direct ourselves for help from the war of Iraq and the events of 9/11 in the World Trade Center, or the stress of a divorce or a relative dying. Running or walking is a healthy, stressful way to instead of smoking, drugs, overeating and drinking alcohol. In an article in March 2003, *Discover* wrote, "As a New Yorker who works in downtown Manhattan, LeDoux has been thinking a lot about these issues since September 11, 2001. Many local residents experienced a conditioned fear response that day, making it hard for them to work in tall buildings or visit the downtown area. LeDoux suspects that traumatic memories will persist in the brains of New Yorkers. The treatment possibilities are not about eliminating the memories so much as restraining the amygdala to respond differently when those memories are triggered." A neuroscience is how battling to subdue the amygdala when those memories hurt the organism. Homocysteine is an amino acid that has high levels of heart disease. Homocysteine acts of several different ways, influencing the development of atherosclerosis. Another theory holds that under stress, our poor diet may cause a rise in blood levels, which has in many foods and also made by the body, similar to cholesterol. Women were designed to prevent heart attacks and strokes, especially, dieting, exercise and weight loss, which reduce to cholesterol and blood pressure. Recommendation with women *and* men are consistent with previous guidelines for healthy bodies.

Exercising is a problem

The problem is that Americans don't like to run... or walk. There is no sidewalk in lots of cases. Outside the front door, there's a six-lane highway between home and the job and the supermarket. Many experts on public health say the way neighborhoods are built is to blame for Americans' physical inactivity, and the resulting epidemic of obesity. The health concern is a new slant on the issue of suburban sprawl, which metro regions have been struggling with for a decade. These health experts bring the deep-pocketed force of private foundations and public agencies into discussions about what neighborhoods should look like. In my suburban house, sidewalks or a bicycle path are not easy to find. In my neighborhood, there is a path to a city park and another one, a county park. But there are not close to shopping centers, restaurants or other neighborhoods. Some people don't like sidewalks in front of their houses. They think it's rural, they don't like sidewalks or streetlights. There are only a few small towns that are easy to walk or bike. There are suburban shopping centers and acres of parking lots. People drive their cars to the malls. Walking or bicycling is an exercise, a hobby... not transportation. In close-to Detroit, one of the most populous cities in the state, Sterling Heights did not have sidewalks. You can bike in the park, but you can't bike from one neighborhood to another. Cars (and trucks and buses) are kings. Beware of busy streets!

A study by the national Centers for Disease Control and Prevention is tracking 8,000 residents of Atlanta to determine whether the neighborhood they live in influences their level of physical exercise. The Robert Wood Johnson Foundation in New Jersey, the country's largest health care philanthropy, is spending $70 million over five years on studies and programs to make it easier for people to walk in suburbs, cities and towns. "We want to engineer routine activity back into people's daily lives," says Kate Kraft, the foundation's senior program officer. "That means we need to start creating more walkable, bikeable communities."

For decades, cities, towns and suburbs have been developed on the assumption that every trip will be made by a car or truck. That has all but eliminated walking from daily life for people in most parts of the country. Americans make fewer than 6% of their daily trips on foot, according to studies by the Federal Highway Administration. Three-quarters of short trips, a mile or less, are made by car, federal studies show. Children don't get much from a workout. Fewer than 13% of students walk to school. That's partly because regulations for school construction effectively encourage that buildings are on large sites at the edge of communities, beyond walking distance for most students, according to a National Trust for Historic Preservation report. Federal health statistics show that nearly 65% of Americans are overweight and that 31% are obese, or more than 30 pounds over a healthy weight. Detroit was No. 1 in obesity in 2004, said a magazine. A big part of the cause is all that driving and not enough walking. Obesity is not just a too-fat lunch or dinner or snacks. We're getting less exercise. People just don't walk that much, if you're live in the suburbs like me. Why you can't walk there from here:

Spread-out neighborhoods. Bigger houses on bigger lots mean neighborhood stretch beyond walking distance for doing errands.

Zoning. Residential neighborhoods are far from jobs and shopping centers, even schools.

Reign of cars. Roads are built big and busy. Intersections and crosswalks are rare. Shopping centers and office parks are set in the middle of big parking lots, all of which have become dangerous places to walk. In many cul-de-sac suburbs and along shopping strips, sidewalks don't even exist.

Cities such as New York, San Francisco and Boston people walk, at least walk to the trains or subways. It's not necessarily for exercise, but simply to get from one place to another. College towns and cities with military bases also have high rates of walking, Census data shows. Houses and workplaces are near each other. If people don't walk to work, they often walk to public transit. In newer cities, especially those in the Sun Belt where growth has boomed since 1950, walking anywhere is not easy. Sometimes, we can't walk or bike or take a bus a job 20-30 miles from our homes. Families wanted more space for their children, so they moved to single-family houses with yards in big residential neighborhoods. Jobs and services, like shopping, followed people to the suburbs, away from the downtown that could easily be served by public transit. But in the hundred years since the paths were laid out, they had fallen into disuse. Instead, people drive down the roads. For my bike, it was carrying behind my car, or my van. The hitch is holding up to four bicycles. It cost me $100. I am always carrying a mountain bike on my van or my car. In and out, the hitch is easy and simple for me. A simple cable lock onto the van and it's one-two-three. When I am close to the park, bike paths, etc. I don't forget my bike because it's already there onto my hitch.

The director of the transportation system in Binghamton, N.Y. ran seminars on pedestrian improvements, paid for by the Robert Wood Johnson Foundation. What we really need to do is redesign our communities so that people walk as a matter of course, the way they used to do, he said. That's a difficult step. "Hopping in your SUV to drive to the park to walk on the trail for 20 minutes and hopping in the car to drive home is not what we need to see." Public health advocates are well-funded allies for advocates of "smart growth," who criticize suburban sprawl and development. They have been arguing for a decade that communities should be walking. Neighborhoods should be built with shorter blocks, smaller yards and streets that connect to each other rather than dead-end. Stores and offices should be close to or mixed with residential neighborhoods.

The Urban Land Institute, a group for developers and planners, estimates that 5% to 15% of new development follows the principles of "walkable" neighborhoods. Nearly 1.6 million homes were built in 2001. The public health experts want to find out what kind of neighborhood designs and amenities have a statistically significant link to increased walking. Some metro areas are taking steps to make their cities pedestrian-friendly, either by upgrading neighborhoods with sidewalks and crosswalks or changing the rules for building developments. The city also made the top 10 "fattest cities" list in the

February 2004 issue of *Men's Fitness* magazine (Detroit was No.1 after Houston, Texas). That may mean Americans don't want to walk regardless of what public health experts urge. Adults, or heath professionals, some don't like to run or walk or golf or play tennis. Think about it. It's why our children don't exercise or even play outside, for the most part.

Stroke victors or victims?

A helpful book is a friend of the stroke victors. These books can be invaluable. In 1981, author and Boston resident Tommye-K. Mayer survived a nearly fatal cerebral hemorrhage. While she survived her stroke, she was left with a paralyzed hand, arm and her left side was paralyzed. She rehabilitated her sufficiently to work full-time and to run a 10K (6.2 miles) race. Her book was "Teaching Me to Run," and also a book, "One-Handed in a Two-Handed World." Tommye-K. Mayer is currently active in Boston's North End neighborhood regarding construction impact on the residents and small businesses, and regarding the historical issue in development. Mayer is also active in the Universal Healthcare movement, as a member of the Massachusetts Ad Hoc Committee to Defend Healthcare. "She had devastating damage to the brain. She was always very motivated, but I didn't think she'd ever be able to do this running. She very pleasantly did not confirm my prognosis," said Dr. Albert Goodgold, New York University Medical Center, a neurologist wrote her book, *"One Step at a Time: Stroke Survivor Overcomes Disabilities."*

"One-Handed in a Two-Handed World" makes it a little easier for survivors.

When they are trying to nail a picture or decorations, their one-handed hammer has a magnet in the head for holding nails. They are difficult and handicapped for a person with one arm and, with my two arms, this tool is a real treasure! There is another tip. There is a plastic clip for using to hold papers with, either for a use for typing or reading, a recipe or instructions, a form or whatever. There are other simple clips even when you have a two-handed world. They can make it improvements from a one-handed world. Correction strips of dispensers, removing or blotting mistakes in a form or a report, can handle correction forms by easily one hand. They can handle correction forms by easily only one hand, displacing the liquid paper that takes a two-handed person with the bottle and a brush on it. A great idea when it comes to forgiving a typo in a letter, or a medical form. A woman, 42, relearned how to write after her stroke six years ago. She rewrote after her rehabilitation six months after it. Recovery was a hard road. You take one step at a time. She owns a car with a left-foot gas pedal and a steering wheel knob that allows her to steer with one hand. She even achieved snow skiing. The relearned the use of one leg ("it doesn't always go where I want.") It took the first three years on the kiddy hill to master this downhill skiing technique. Now, she skis on the intermediate slope.

Mary, who I know from aphasia meetings, owns a van. Even though she doesn't drive, it's hers – a personal van that carries her and her wheelchair. She asks everyone to drive her on the van and its accessible wheelchair. A push to the button and opens its doors, lowering the ramp. A personal chauffeur is happy to drive with her accessible personal van to grocery stores, movies and shopping malls. Mary uses her electrical battery wheelchair and she is looooong gone!

All of these things, one single small idea, has it makes it easier, especially one with a wheelchair or a disabled arm or hand. Reading is visually large print, a handy for everyone. Reader's Digest and a few other magazines, paperbacks and best sellers are published large print. "Teaching me to run," Mayer wrote. "In mid-sentence he stepped away from me, deeper into the center of my living room, not focused so much on the movement as on his thought and the words he'd chosen to express it. I'm not sure he was even aware he'd moved. Me? I was watching as much as listening. Watching and noticing. It was different now, the way he moved – smooth, more fluid, more confident. It was almost as if, after thirty-five years of living in his body, he'd discovered its extent, and understood that extent now too; understanding the parameters of its parts, internalizing as well, the purposes for each of those parts. It was as if before, his body had been only packaging for his brain, unworthy of his consideration as long as it continued to get what his brain needed and to move his brain where it needed to be. 'It's strange, you know,' he was saying, 'most of the time I really hate running. I have to make myself get out there and do it.'"

I ran a mile in my neighborhood. I ran 10 miles to the park. I didn't have to relearn to running or walking, without a cane or a walker. I'm fortunate. I ran twice a week in winter (indoors whenever I can), four or five times outdoors in the spring, fall and summer seasons. I wrote and ran. I ran to my travels and business at the beaches in Florida, in mountains in Colorado, in urban cities like San Francisco and Chicago. I tried to run at employees at Business News Publishing. I tried to coerce people who were playing and working at conventions or business conferences or meetings. Before breakfast, at lunch, and after dinner – whenever, where ever. It makes it easier for packing one pair of running shoes, along with running shorts and a tee shirt. If I can, I will use a small cassette player and earphones, for the music while I am running. I have a cassette with the movie's song "Rocky", "L.A. Woman," by the Doors, "Born to Run," and "Glory Days" by Bruce Springsteen, "Got Me Under Pressure by Z.Z. Topp, "Rebel Yell" by Billy Idol, "Burnin' Hell" by John Lee Hooker, "Promises in the Dark" by Pat Benetar, and "Locomotive Train" by Jethro Hull, a few of my favorites. Classical, blues, jazz, even radio for talking to news or sports hums a long, long distance and hours.

"Running wherever and whenever I chose to take it," Mayer said. "But especially I remembered running on the beach, on the hard-packed, sandy beach at low-tide in front of my folks' house. Even after ten years, sometimes I still dreamt . . . 'What do you suppose it is?' David asked. We sat down to eat. And to talk more. 'It,' I said, dragging myself from my reverie, trying to recall his last remark, and then remembering. 'The feeling you could go on forever?' 'Yes,' he said, the next forkful poised to eat. 'I couldn't, of course. There's a limit to how far the human body can run before it wears out.'" I never had to quit running, unlike Mayer. I never had to slow, or ease myself. There was a lot of warm, sunny running days (or outside snowy, freezing days in the YMCA), in my life. I thought of another 10 miles at the Crim race in August 23, 2003. That was just a year (14 months) from my stroke. I was a lot of quicker races than I was running 10 years ago but not 20 years, when I was age 29. I'm not trying to become 29. That's not my objection. I really wanted to run at the age of 49. That was my whole goal. My time: around 8 minutes per mile. The same, even better, than my running before my stroke.

Ernie Harwell, 85, the ex-Detroit Tigers baseball announcer, has been walking every daily, from 30 years. I met him in 2003 and he's a great talker and a superb speaker. He retired after age 80, when he was in the announcing box. Harwell can talk about a baseball player and the baseball team last year and 50 years ago. His trademarks are almost little sentences: "That's a loooong ball, a home run!" and "He watched the fastball by him like it was a barn door." He and wife Lulu, 83, have long built walking into their lives in other ways. In 2003, Harwell was at the age of 85! I saw him when he was speaking at my St. Rene Church. He had a lifting language and he was convincing to many others. And he looks good! He is shorter, but his voice is larger. He talked about baseball and players – yesterday and a half-century ago – and talked about his life. I wished I could talk to Harwell, and have the same energetic days with him. Do you don't have the time to walk or run? Showed that walking at a moderate pace as little as an hour a week halved the risk of heart disease for a group of women and older. Some experts suggest more physical activity makes a half an hour or hour a day. But for people who normally don't exercise, minutes a day can make a difference. One out of four Americans report they do not have consistently physical activity.

Take some time; look at your expectations and limitations honestly, before you run or bicycle. Set some talking goals: practice short sentences or phases describing some feature of your life, from three months from now, one year from now and three years from now. "To stimulate your imagination, describe each of these stages it might relate to children, career changes, family income, religious involvement, etc." recommends *Divorce and Beyond.* Here are some suggestions to help you run and realize your goals:

- List all the things that you want out of life. Ask yourself:Is this really my goal? (Not a 10-K run or a mile when starting.)
- Am I too afraid of past experiences to give it a fair try?
- Will I know when I have reached my goal? (Not a contest, as a determine.)
- Is the goal worth the struggle? (Is it too hard; maybe you'll *hate* it if it was too hard.)
- Is the goal realistic, given my schedule, finances, and talents as well as possible opposition from others?
- Organize your goals in the order of their importance. Don't try to run a 26.2 miles marathon. You'll be too tired, and too drained to really attempt to make a run or a race.
- Work out specific things you can do to achieve your goals. Talk with others, and don't be afraid to ask for help.
- Choose these goals with activities that can be started immediately (some goals may have to wait for a while). Make them short-termed enough so that you can achieve them with ease.
- Make sure that your goals are clear, specific, measurable, and realistic.

You'll like it if you run with friends or a group. Or if you have a scenic, pretty place (outside, not just inside a gym or your basement), a park or on a walking/bicycling trail or path. Maybe two times a gymnasium or a track or stationary bicycle but make sure it's a certain picturesque scene, every week or every two weeks. Your times will be hard at the gym and inside, and will be better at the outside in the park.

Careers, or time for a job?

"Language is much more than words. It involves our ability to recognize and use words and sentences. Much of this capability resides in the left hemisphere of the brain, and when a person has a

stroke or other type of injury that affects the left side of the brain, it typically disrupts their ability to use language."
Anastasia Ramer, PhD, CCC-SLP
StrokeConnection May/June 2003

In 1975, I was at Wayne State University in Detroit. I got a bachelor of liberal arts and a major in journalism. There was no doubt, I would be a reporter or a writer. I began a freelancer, and still I am a freelancer, with a book on the subject, aphasia. I never wanted nor wished with a job as a speech language pathologist or a researcher or an occupational therapist. I yearn for writing general communications to the public. But I had aphasia after my stroke. When I wanted a job, it was suggested as a hospital volunteer. That is not the same. What I want is with a writer, not just as any job. I take ideas and put them onto paper. It's not with taking patients with tests, or copying cases. Volunteering is one thing, having a job is another. I was at my mid-career. Moving, up to the mountain. I started as an intern (the college newspaper, the South End) next a part time or as a freelance newspaper. It was my first job almost 30 years ago. It was almost slave wages, but it wasn't volunteering either. I earned money, maybe $20 or $30 per story, $5 or $10 for individual photographs. I had my camera and developed the photographs in the darkroom too, black and white film. They didn't have any digital cameras. There were photo papers and a "wet" darkroom chemicals (I can still smell the fixer). At a long time, 20 years from my journalism career, I started as a trade magazine – ensconced in our individual offices, in our own computers. It really was a concept! In newspapers, you shared a desk, computer, even a phone. There are also cubicles, but I had my own office. I continued as an editor and for 10 years I got another job, as a publisher. There were incentives, in sales and equaled the dollars/number of pages, or pages/number of ads. We were successful. We were a real "family" among our advertisers and our readers, and our clique of writers. We went into their sheet metal shops with notebooks and cameras. They were generous and they were happy and proud with their trades. We asked and learned what they did. It was a community newspaper but a national trade magazine also. It was the top of the roller coaster, making it in the late 1990s and early 2000s. There were very prosperous business days in the United States. Just when my brain had a sudden sleeping attack.

Some individuals with aphasia return to work. However, most are forced to retire or change jobs and work in a modified capacity. There are very few jobs that do not require speech and language skills. Think about it. Individuals with mild or even moderate aphasia are sometimes able to return to work, but often with some changes in job responsibilities and a reduced workload. Recovery is a slow process that usually requires a minimum of a year of treatment, including helping the individual and family understand and adjust to long term deficits. Many patients continue to show improvements years after their strokes. When formal speech therapy ends, informal aphasia support groups are proving beneficial. These groups are starting to increase the numbers and accessibility. When a part of the heart or the brain succumbs, a heart attack or stroke occurs. Inflammation can also cause certain plaques to rupture the vessels. Blood clots tend to form over ruptured plaques and can then occlude arteries, leading to such atherosclerotic complications as heart attack and stroke. Doctors feel that a lifestyle modification, such as running, can be a form of cardiovascular prevention.

Is your career can be really "retired"? I hope not. I'm only 49. But when I am retired to my career? I don't know, that's the thing. I hope I can write an article, a book, when I am 69 or 79 or 89. Provide us with a detailed description of your daily routine, according to MetLife Insurance Company, a personal profile. Everything? How detailed a description? (They have you 2 ½ spaces, like this:

Is that enough? Is it too detailed… or not? What time do you get in the morning? The same as I go to work, at 6:30 or 7 a.m. When do you go to bed? 11:00 or 11:30 p.m. Does that matter? What's the difference, anyway? Do you sleep or toss and turn? Why? Again, does that matter? Have your sleeping habits changed since your condition(s) began? Please explain. I didn't change any of my sleeping habits. Even when I had a job at 8:30 a.m. my lifestyle went on. Except sleeping alone, without sex with my wife. Should I tell them? They didn't ask me with sex, they simply asked sleeping. It's a big, nasty ex-marriage and a divorce. There is always a big, nasty ex-marriage and a divorce, isn't it? There was always an "incident," never just a divorce. Do they understand, or comprehend, or gossip about my lifestyle? Do they care, or maybe not? Have there been any changes in your ability to care for your personal needs and grooming? Please. I wear the same shirt every day and cut my hair every five years or so. I bite my fingernails and don't brush my teeth. Next question? Have you thought about killing yourself and/or your employees? That's a true question, honest. Am I crazy or stupid? When do you expect to return to your job/occupation either on a full-time or part-time basis? It's easy. I expect to be there the next day. Do I really, honestly, expect a job? Nope. It'll be a little longer. How long? Two years, three years or five years. I don't know. I DON'T KNOW do you get the picture? Do you feel you could return to your job/occupation if accommodations were made? Maybe, if I had a secretary. They can translate. They can say, "That's Ed and he's my boss and he doesn't speak." If I can speak, or I can write I can have my job... maybe. It's a long, two or three years after rehabilitating your workplace. Your new employees probably don't know you. Your face was familiar with your older employees and they ask, "What wrong with Ed?" after two years or three years or five years. You don't have your job, don't have your desk, and don't have an office. Believe it or not.

"When I opened up Snips (snips is a tool for cutting the metal ducts and was a trades magazine) this week, I was shocked when I read your note," said one reader, another contractor. "I readily had no idea that you were out for these last months with your stroke." He and a friend were running at a national convention. "...Next year I promise to be in better shape; I know you'll be up for it, and we will resume an early morning run..." said one writer.

"I read with great interest your 'note' in the February (2003) issue and was pleased to learn of your progress. It is clear that you *have* been faced with an uphill run like none before," said a letter from an association regarding my job. They're a great people, and I would be sorry for their communion. "... We extend only our best wishes for your continued success and good health," she wrote. I wish her, and the people she represents, own their hopes and successes, always.

New Horizons

New Horizons is a private, not-for-profit organization founded in 1964 that began as an outgrowth of a parent's group concerned with the lack of opportunities available for people with disabilities. Today, it has grown to branches and numerous work sites in the community. It's a United Way agency, approved by the Bureau of Worker's Disability Compensation, certified as an employment agency. They have:
Employment services
Employment services coordination
Employment transition services
Comprehensive vocational evaluation services
Employee development services, etc.

They'll develop an individual support plan that includes employment goals and address all pertinent issues regarding SSI and SSDI benefits, as well as assisting in the job search and help find job leads. They do not pay a placement fee and are not a placement agency. They can be available on site to help you with a transition period. Be determined. They have a lot of cases. I took a number, almost another 6-8 weeks to talk to me. After tests and registration (and more papers) they have sloo-ooow to get a counselor. I was not important to them, I thought, just a number. I seldom see my counselor. I called them, once or twice. Two weeks were in common, three or four weeks or almost two months getting my "rehabilitation coordinator" at my "career development." "Take therapy," I was told. "You have Blue Cross. See a psychologist about your depression." Depressed, who me? I wasn't despondent or depressed. I wanted a job, maybe my last one, and I wanted my speech. They do "handle" employer expectations, resume preparation, applications and references, and career explorations. They have the following: CAD operators, courtesy clerks, data entry clerks, sales associates, child care staff, engineers, restaurant staff, etc. Engineers? They mean low minimum wages: custodians, janitors, sanitation, dishwashers, retail store clerks, etc. I can read the classifieds. I can read a Help Wanted flyer or announcement. I can write my resume. Rehabilitation counselors create a familiar environment with clients had a brain injury. Don't expect them to help persons with aphasia. The counselors aren't specialists. Don't expect them to find your own job. You MUST get one. You will have to read the classifieds, fax, email or make the job interviews for yourself. Do be honest about the illness and/or injury. Do NOT over encourage such as "You'll be all right. You'll be back to work in no time." Don't jot your age in a resume or application. That's not their business, whether you're 40 or 60. If you are retired, or disabled, keep the last job on your resume. For example, keep your dates from your job from you first got it: 1990 – or don't close the date from your last job, if you can help it. You're still there on the paperwork, right? Don't say you were looking for a job the last five years. It sounds like you're a loser. Don't say you were fired or because you were not able to work your job. Do NOT tease or encourage the interviewer to say inappropriate words. Do laugh with the person when appropriate. Do end each visit on a positive note. Do NOT use one-word statements like "Relax!" This may cause anger, resentment, and agitation. Do NOT rely on what the person says he/she can do. Do remember the person may laugh or cry easily (their words, not mine – that's a little disheartening.) Do remember that no two people are alike. Do NOT compare.

The state career development has the right to evaluate eligibility. They must obtain information to verify you have impairment and give information that can be obtained from you, your family members, physician or therapist. You will be notified of this eligibility decision, continually re-evaluated are services to you may be discontinued if it appears they will not help you to become employed. If you are found eligible for services, you have the right to obtain written information about options available to you in preparing your Individualized Plan for Employment. You have the right to obtain help from a counselor. More than 70% of people with disabilities are unemployed. How often your case is reviewed depends on the severity of your condition. The frequency can range from six months to seven years. Here are general guidelines:

Improvement expected – if medical improvement can be predicted when benefits start, your first review should be six to 18 months later.

Improvement possible – if medical improvement is possible but cannot be predicted, your case will be reviewed about every three years.

Improvement not expected – if medical improvement is not likely, your case will be reviewed only about once every five to seven years.

(From Social Security – *What You Need to Know When You Get Disability Benefits*.)

The act is PABSS: Protection and Advocacy for Beneficiaries of Social Security, a part of the Work & Work Incentives Improvement Act of 1999. In the act, it is helping people with disabilities to return to work. The PABSS Advocate and the Attorney provide the following services:

Information and referral
Advice and advocacy
Technical assistance
Mediation and legal representation
Education and training
Learning for a career

Don't be afraid to enroll for college classes. No time for having classes? Please. You probably have a lot of time: eight hours from your job, after you retired or were disabled. Polly Perez, a stroke survivor, she was a nurse, speaker and author of "Brain Attack." She said, "… I spent two and a half hours in the hospital business office discussing my bill, which seems to be getting larger and larger... The second change in our income knocked me for a loop. In some respects, I feel that I'm responsible for our money problems. If I hadn't had the brain attack…" She had two speaking engagements, then another, and so on. "Since I can't speak from notes, I had to write out the words to every one of my speeches…"

But if you're 40, 60 or 80, get interested. Get a career development: computer typing/keyboarding; computer graphics; email, websites and Internet (you can register your own Internet Domain Name); Excel including spreadsheets and analyzing numeric information; administrative assistants; builders licensing; medical terminology; positioning your investments; accounting principles; French, Italian and German perhaps; and English as a second language.

Helpful hints for returning adults:

Plan early for your return to school. Meet with a counselor first thing when you come to campus. Counselors can offer assistance in planning your educational and career goals. Take advantage of early registration. This will give you a better chance to get the courses you want at the times that are convenient for you. Know your strengths and weaknesses. Work to improve your weak areas. Take full advantage of student services on campus. Counselors can direct you to financial aid, tutoring services and job placement.

Encourage yourself! Don't expect to be perfect. Build your aphasia support group. Meet and study with other aphasia survivors. Choose a place to study a quiet place. After aphasia you don't need talking, t.v.'s or phoning when you study your subject.

Don't be afraid if you're retired even if you're 65 or 75 or 85. Take a dance class: tap, ballet, jazz, swing and country (plus technihop, whatever that means). Kickboxing? Yoga? Karate? All of them. Hypnosis for weight loss or stop smoking, heart saver first aid and adult CPR, and anger management with stress releaser. Public school districts or community college makes them handier and easier to get to your classes. Chances are, you have a class or seminar close to your backyard. The universities as a national research learning a teaching and service mission. It fosters creativity and strives for excellence in performance and exhibition. It recognizes its obligation to serve. It strives to serve the disciplines and professions represented among its academic programs as well as public and privates sector organizations and associations at local, state, and national levels.

I received a scholarship with Camp Cavell from the National Stroke Association (NSA), an American Heart Association, in summers near Lexington, Mich. A weekend of friends and good food, with swimming, games, bonfire-singing, and activities depending on the stroke. Camp Cavell is a YWCA camp. It has cabins with seven to nine campers and one counselor. They have cabins with electricity, heat, bathrooms and showers, with four-inch mattresses – hardly a rough-style camping! Alcoholic beverages and illegal drugs are not permitted at camp. Smoking is not encouraged. Meals and programs are planned from Friday evening until brunch on Sunday. They have food aplenty and snacks, and they plan low-fat meals. Not elegant, but stick-to-your-ribs. "This is your weekend, so feel free to participate in the activities of your choice." It's on beautiful Lake Huron, one of the Great Lakes. I heard from Camp Cavell at while a meeting at aphasia. People can be a source of information, not just social conversations.

"We had volunteers on-hand to assist with the care-giving needs of a stroke survivor, if needed," explained Beth Pfalzgraf of Novi, Michigan, co-chair of the retreat and volunteer. "This retreat can offer many families a chance to vacation again in the safety of a specialized environment and gives primary caregivers a much-needed break."

The Stroke Connection Retreat was the brainchild of Pfalzgraf, Sheila Daley of Grosse Pointe Woods and fellow co-chair of the retreat and Lisa Choate of the American Heart Association in response to a need for stroke survivors and their caregivers to experience a fun activity like camping. The trio readily acknowledges that the camp can only thrive with the efforts of volunteers from area hospitals, stroke support groups, therapists and others who donate their time. For information about attending next year's Stroke Connection Retreat, for contact the American Heart Association at 800-968-2425.

The Columbus Writers Conference has a two-day conference at Columbus, Ohio. It's 300 miles from me, but that's not a problem. Writers' conference can be a useful for writers, suggested at ads and articles at *Writer's Digest*, a monthly magazine published every month (12 months a year). See their magazine or their web site: http/www.-writersdigest.com. It's one or several conferences of almost every state in the calendar. More than 35 different presentations are by writers, editors and literary agents. "Corporate climate" says the corporate environment and why it is a boon to writers. "Bulldog tactics" says a 12-step process for turning your passion into a successful publishing experience. Don't write it only once, get a sharp eye and not just by your friends or relatives. At one-to-one consultations and a critique are offered, at a reasonable price from $150 to $250, some of them have scholarships. Novel writing, non-fiction writing, creative, freelance, short stories, "secrets to a successful publishing career", marketing, scripts, plays, getting (or firing) an agent, writing for Hollywood, science fiction, Romantics, children's books, poetry, etc. It can be truly chutzpah for networking. Don't be a wallflower. Don't be at a dance and don't be a non-dancer. The agents were there to talk with them. Oakland University, Rochester, Mich., had a writers' conference annually. It is every October and is just minutes from my house. I feel that anything within 300 miles is not too far driving. That means Columbus, Ohio to me, and big cities (and big universities) from Chicago to Toronto to Cleveland, etc. That is a single day of driving. Writing is for everyone to keep a journal and keeping memos for the life of post-stroke. If nothing, it's touching and poignant for yourself and your loved ones.

The three job stressors are absenteeism, accidents and alcoholism. The three areas are your own reactions, your support network and your employee. Recognize that when stress is involved. The Male Stress Survival Guide by Georgia Witkin, PhD, suggested "encourage his participation is stress burn-off techniques – both physical activity and emotional outlets. And don't forget the healing properties of laughter. Look for opportunities to laugh together." Behavioral early warning signs are observable, repetitive, and usually consistent for each person, they are potentially the most useful of all early warning signals for the beginnings of male stress. Six months, have been the way of life, the way it has been before aphasia – a point of reference. Before the stroke, and after the stroke. It's time to realign myself. The hospital aligned my tires. You're discouraged that recovery hasn't been faster and more complete. It's time to hurt. You begin to sense that improving is not going to be faster. You have shown that life is not the same life anyway. The rate of change is beginning to slow. You must reassure that value is the best. Some performance is far below that pre-stroke. I can read it, a little than write it, but I can't just a task of conversation. Two, three words amid sentences, but not 10 or 12 or 15. It takes some years to talk a full conversation (never, maybe) and I feel that I'm sad or disappointed because of that. I'm also sad because a historic study shows that almost 50% of people have had recurrent strokes. Fifty million people worldwide have strokes or TIAs (mini-strokes) annually. A study has revealed that over 500,000 of those incidents annually could be prevented by using a combination of perindopril (a high-blood pressure medication) and indapamide (a diuretic). The trials found that using ACEON® (generically known as perindopril), an ACE inhibitor in combination with a diuretic, reduced the risk for secondary stroke by as much as 50%. There was a 38% reduction in fatal strokes in patients using the perindopril-based therapy. In addition, there was up to a 50% reduction in stroke-related dementia and serious cognitive impairment for TIA patients who went on to experience a recurrent stroke. PROGRESS showed even patients with normal blood pressure would benefit from this therapy.

The 6,000-patient trial, the first randomized trial to use an ACE inhibitor or combination ACE inhibitor and diuretic, was conducted in 10 countries over the past five years. According to a test by investigators, "These results are the biggest single advance in secondary stroke prevention." Patti Shwayder, NSA executive director/CEO said, "National Stroke Association (NSA) believes the American public needs to know this information and work with their health care providers to do all they can to prevent strokes." According to NSA, secondary strokes are fatal in 25% of the cases, and often result in greater disability. On average, they are also more expensive to treat than the first strokes. Studies show that within five years of a stroke, 24% of women and 42% of men will experience another stroke. ACEON is currently approved by the U.S. Food and Drug Administration for use an anti-hypertensive (blood pressure lowering) medication. The drug is classified as an angiotensin converting enzyme (ACE) inhibitor. ACE inhibitors maintain the elasticity of the blood vessel wall, protecting it from damage and decreasing the likelihood of blood clots or hemorrhage. The perindopril-based therapy results were seen in addition to aspirin.

Resources for talking

Don't be afraid from talking. It's not easy, I know. My student therapy said, "Mr. Bas is a trouble maker." She was kidding, I think. But it's true. I'm a barkin' dog. It sounds like a rusted wheel. My letter to MetLife said: "I am disappointed with your insurance." Or "I am disappointed in your Denial Notice. As defined by my Group Plan, 'total disability means that because of a sickness or an injury: 1) You can not do your job and 2) You can not do any other job for which you are fit by your education, your training or your experience.'" Let them know, that you are disappointed. Don't say you're angry. They don't like that. They're afraid from you, or ignore you. Don't be scary, but say persistent and obstinate. Let them hear, or let third party suggest what you are saying. Your therapist can speak for yourself, maybe your doctor will send a letter for you. Don't be a pest or a nuisance, but let them you're stubborn. Tell them once, or twice, and forget about it. "He'll be better if he can take a class from speech language," said one doctor. Tell them, that you'll be better with classes – not now, not yesterday, but maybe in a year, or two years.

Communications is a two-lane road. I took a communication class for talking my own two teenagers, but how to talk with others and hear from children to their adults? How does your child usually respond? How do they feel? For some, a child is talking either a goal for some attention, power, revenge or a display of inadequacy. They talk with words are angry, feeling either threatened or from a hopeful sense. You can build a good relationship with your children by showing respect, having fun, giving encouragement or showing love. Don't expect them with talking teenagers every single day. They won't feel like talking. Being a parent is a stressful job. Breathe deeply for about 15 minutes, suggested authors "The Parent's Handbook." Let your normal breathing pace. Don't force it. Quietly say "calm" as you breathe in, and say "down" as you breathe out. Do this until you feel relaxed. Reduce stress and create a pleasant emotional state by beginning by tensing your hands into fists, then relaxing them. Learn how muscle tension feels so you can relax a tense feeling. Accept yourself, they said. "Every day, accept yourself and take time to concentrate on your positive qualities. Make self-affirming statements, like 'I'm learning to become more effective,' or 'I'm growing more confident.'" Give them a letter, a card with your comments (Congratulations! with a report card), emails, a brief note, and so on.

Don't be afraid to ask a girl or a woman for a date. You don't want to ask her, right? Maybe she doesn't like you. But maybe she will. I didn't like it. The truth is it's uncomfortable when you have a stutter or a falter with words or you can't say it without a complete sentence. She said that she couldn't date with me, because she was dating a boyfriend. But wasn't that better than she didn't like me/like my speech/like I was too short? Plenty of people have a stroke in their families or friends. Speech isn't a serious catastrophe. If you type, email is much better. A realtor (she) was that I was e-mailing for every couple of days or so, buying my condo and selling my house. It took me a lot of time. After yet another email, I wanted to take her a non-business dinner at a local restaurant. My email was pretty good, at least I think – the wording and grammar was really not so bad. I wrote a sentence, then read it aloud at first, and a second time or a third. You can do it: email before you have it "Send" for him/her. Do the spell checker on your computer. Or get a paperback dictionary/thesaurus. I got a tape recorder for the reason for this book. I was reading aloud, and it smoothed the wording for the book. Another close friend, a woman, was living in my condo project. I saw her and she was walking, almost every day. I said, "You want to walk?" and she said, "Sure!" It was five words that involved a close relationship. I can always say four words.

It seems like every aphasic survivor wants to understand everyone with all the details from their stroke. "I had a stroke... 17 years, three months, two days, eight hours and 17 minutes ago." They want you to understand everything, realize all the minute details. The hospitalization, the family, where you had it, the doctors and nurses, the operation and all the medical personnel and their names, the diet, exercise, and so on. Grandparents will wear a sweatshirt that says: "Ask me about my grandchildren!" They should wear a shirt: "Ask me about my aphasia!" I really don't like the details. Do you? Maybe one or two, but the hospitalization and doctors, that's too much! Nobody doesn't want to tell you on the theory of stroke, either.

Talk. How do I do it? I don't, but try to continue to look for resources outside the home that might provide some communication stimulation, said *Coping with Aphasia* by Jon G. Lyon. "Having the outside world be more receptive to interacting with your loved one, and making new friends are not the same thing," Lyon said. My three best tips I have included:

A friend or family. I am at ease with their talking. Like my sisters, or close friends. When she/he talks, and I am familiar with them I can communicate. She knows how I talk, and some times will prompt my conversations.

Short subjects, to where I can talk – a little. A phone call, a salesman or the woman telling me the new phone bill said, "Is this Edward Bas?" "Yes, it's Ed Bas," I respond. For example: What is the question? It's a short answer and it's a brief conversation.

The regular, really tough sentences. I try to email them. I try not to telephone them. When I have to phone, I write down on paper. Sometimes the person to understand my questions or my doubts, or they understand I had a stroke or aphasia. Talk slowly.

It doesn't get better

Asked if I was going to Wayne State for its speech therapy in the coming semester, I was trying a reason to end it. I wasn't that keen at WSU's beginning classes in speech therapy. Stroke survivor Paul Sage was surprised. "Well, it's just a life that is good and bad. One day that is a good therapy, and sometimes therapy that is bad." True, good or bad, one day at a time. That's like therapy, classes, friends, driving, jobs, and life. You've sounded all the right words. The correct sentences, "and" "but" with chain links, conjunctions and associations. You are so painful for your speech it would hopefully take an aspirin to end a headache. Will I even talk better, or with a "real" conversation – better than two or three or four words, or gestures, or people who will finish your conversations? I've talked to people who had strokes 15, 20, 25 years ago. That's a long time. But 25 years isn't a long life. Can it get better? Fuck it, I thought. It doesn't get better or worse.

"The Land God Forgot" is a poem by Robert Service. He wrote about the 1850s in his life in the Yukon: the whiteness of the coldness and the soulness of the silence. The soulness that I have of aphasia, with its cold, forbidding silence. A displaced Englishman he penned the immense Canadian Yukon. It was as different as he could be a pioneer or a gold miner, not a British gentleman. You can hear ears straining. You can hear an ounce, or miles of quietness. So loud with your loud talking, and your yelling and screaming. Your own voice can summon an avalanche. A smooth, white blanket, it had a fog or snowing around you. "The lonely sunsets flare forlorn, Down valleys dreadly desolate; The lordly mountains soar is scorn, As still as death, as stern as fate." A silence so loud it is deafening. A hush soundness of mind, a light noise, a pin dropped at a whisper at temperatures 30 below. An affinity I have one. A sound as quiet, as it can be at times, it can reverberate like an avalanche. Not unlike the affection of wintry Yukon, the white blanket is used as aphasia – it's more like an alliance. A friendly white wintry blanket: "So gaunt against the gibbous moon, Piercing the silence velvet-piled, A lone wolf howls his ancient rune – The fell arch-spirit of the Wild... Let the lone wolf-cry all express. The hate insense of thy hand, Thy heart's abysmal loneliness." You can do it. Scream the words! Let the lone wolf-cry all express... Thy heart's (and brain's) abysmal loneliness...succumb all silence, quiet and gaunt and scorn. Barkin' dog!

Overture

It's a tough, unyielding, mean life. Don't forget talking, don't forget arguing either. Make them listen! I don't try to be a barking dog. Sometimes a dog can bark just to say, "I'm here! Pet me or pay attention to me." A barkless dog doesn't have focus around him. In a year after you can survive from your stroke, it's better but it isn't perfect or even achieved. But it's important, to everyone understand what it takes aphasia and why it's a handicap. Try to telephone with a utility: the telephone, electric, and the gas company. Try and tell them what you want. Call the insurance company or cable t.v. company, if you have to. Don't yell or frustrated. Tell them what it's like. If you live in a house or apartment, you need to have a phone – now what? Try to place a phone number at the utilities about maybe the first or second or third caller. Without speaking with aphasia, but it's not impossible. You should not be ashamed. You can do it. Get a job, classes, money (funding, wages, etc.), what it takes for an exercise, a diet or drugs. It doesn't take a minute, or an hour, or a day.

Aphasia is not a simple operation, or a simple therapy. It's harder and tougher. It takes years and lots of work. My life is before-stroke and after-stroke. It's true. Any people will say it. I pretended it is not true. I had a class from the county, Community Assessment Referral & Education (CARE) is dedicated to the prevention of alcohol, tobacco and other drug abuse. It was about my communication with my teenagers. My two teenagers are not into alcohol or drugs. As a beginning of the seminar told the message: "Until society views the drug problem as a public and social problem rather than a moral failure rather than a moral failure, we will make headway in promoting the health and public safety of our citizens." It told children about goals, beliefs, and attention. It told us that communications are valuable. I say that communications is a lonely, dreadful life. I can spell Hippocrates or explain Broca's brain, but I can't readily think the words "from" and "with" – two little, ugly words introduced into my conversations. It has been simulated since that day of the stroke. It's not a way that is normal. It's a real change of life, if not a common one. A therapist told me, it's every day, maybe as long as a lifetime. It's different with me, he said. My speech therapist told me has a dilemma. It's hard for him to write with correct spelling. I cringe when I see him write recieve rather than receive. I read his writing and it's *terrible!* You can't write novels or magazine articles, can't even write letters and emails – maybe– with inaccurate spelling. A friend wrote in my emails, *I had a devorce last year.* I stopped and had to reread it. He was trying to say, that he had a divorce with his wife. It took me a while. I know at least two of those friends who cannot spell. It's hard but not impossible, like aphasia. My speech therapist said, it's a long life, and probably won't get better despite the classes and studies and dictionaries (thank god for spell checker in computers!) A few of them who can't spell or write, but also don't read. Newspapers, magazines, books, novels – none of them. And they can get by. They can read, they say; they just don't like reading!

I am almost two years after my post-stroke. I'm trying to take classes, maybe even scholarships or the state rehabilitation services. I'm into physical: running, bicycling, volleyball, tennis, golf, bowling, downhill skiing and cross country skiing, sometimes from friends, sometimes alone. I took a six-week seminar on communication, really about my teenagers. It's from the county government or the probate court supposed to handle your families. They are one of many of agencies serving kids with drugs or alcohol. With my son and daughter don't want to drugs or alcohol. But I have a problem: communication. Or aphasia, exactly. The classes don't hurt, I thought. They are helping me. A suggestion from the psychologist who gives the seminar in the first day says, "Do you need this class? Of course! It helps in helping to communicate, especially with you and you and you! All of us, I believe.

Your life is changing with a stroke. It is different. It's not having a heart attack; having a stroke is a year, two years, or more. One person told me, aphasia is four years from his stroke. He said, a day from his life was better. His life was almost dead, as he called it. He quit driving a car, and his days are viewing movies in his television. It could have been worse. He tells me, it's good and understanding even with his stuttering problem. A medicine is a day-to-day ending from a stroke, but does not help with aphasia. The same awful technology and neurons last every day, amid a speech-language therapy. "Communication is part of our everyday life," told Debra Busacco of the American Society Heart Association. "As we age there may be some normal changes in speech, language, swallowing, and hearing that may affect our ability to communicate effectively. It is important to understand which changes are part of the normal aging process and which communication changes may warrant further evaluation by as ASHA-certified speech-language pathologist or audiologist." Be aware of communication. Writing or reading, not just talking, changes are part of the stroke. Don't let it get a hopeless time or life. Whether if it takes me two years, or five years, or 10 years, give it a chance. Don't give it time. Use your speaking. Do a barking dog. Make sense and yell or shout – emphatically, loudly! Good luck... and have a healthy life.

"Remember, 'I am alive.' It could have turned out differently."
From The Stroke Group at Mercy Hospital
Iowa City, Iowa

Chapter 6

Postmortem

On day, November 15, 2003, I was dead. That is a bad analogy. I was not breathing, said nurses at the intensive care unit, and had not a pulse. One nurse didn't have a pulse, and she would sense it – they were, after all, ICU medical personnel. I had an accident at Oakwood Hospital in Dearborn, Mich. visiting (or observing, really) my mother. She was a patient at the hospital. She was dying from bladder cancer. She died two days from then in November 2003. It was early morning: 1:30 a.m. I thought, if people are suffering a heart attack or stroke, it's better at a hospital, accompanied by plenty of nurses and doctors. There were at least seven or eight of them in the hallway when I crashed – literally. It's a word: syncope. The definition is a blackout, or a coma, resulting insufficient blood flow to the brain. I didn't have a heart attack. I didn't think so, anyway. I was light headed, a little queasy and nauseous. I was unconscious within two minutes. I wasn't dying, really. One nurse told me, "We were worried! You were as white as a sheet!" I had a little complicated setback for more things after having a stroke. I was angry. Not scared. I did have plenty of time after my stroke to get my things to me and my family. I wanted to get a job, get to the meetings and classes, drive my van for my daughter's classes, etc. I only had a blackout for a minute or two minutes. Life and death at those times is defined within six minutes. That's how long rescuers have to get the heart started for the victim to survive.

The goal is to get chest compressions started immediately after a cardiac-arrest victim collapses and to keep the compressions going until medical employees can arrive.

During this time, the blood in the brain and other vital organs still has oxygen that was picked up when it last passed through the lungs before the heart stopped. The body needs chest compressions to keep this blood moving.

There was a male nurse gave me cardiopulmonary respiration (CPR). There isn't a chance for the patient to get him awake or consciousness. They actually have only a minute or two minutes, without a pulse or breathing. He was a gorilla, banging his fists into my heart! It hurt like hell, like on thumping a hardball by a Tigers pitcher. I was carried on the emergency level from the hospital; lots of tests, blood pressure, ekgs, echo, sugar, etc. I felt fine. The tests were normal. It cost me a lot of money. I am grateful I had health insurance. The doctor said, "We'll look at you for this night before we'll let you stay for the next day." It was 12 hours from my "heart attack." It was only 8 a.m.! From another doctor, the second recommend, said four hours from then that I was fine, and I could leave before 1 p.m. Thank you! I said it, and again. I walked quickly. I had two bad cases from my hospital (lots of pricks with needles, but that's minor): an open wound at my right temple where I fell (looked gross, but it wasn't bad at all) on the tile hallway; and the compression from my male nurse (a big hard fist!) He performed CPR and the compression bruised me a couple of days from then. If you never had compressing of your heart with an ICU male nurse, you're lucky! I'm thinking, was it really a close to my death or did I have just a fainting or unconscious? He was trying to give me CPR, so I was very grateful. Two days from then I had a stress test with my cardiologist: ok. "The patient is a 40 year old male, who was admitted to the hospital about 1 or 1:30 (a.m.) He was on the Third Floor visiting his mother, who was dying. He was standing in the hall talking with his sisters. He said he was tired and he was stressed, and he was suddenly felt dizzy and fell to the floor. He had a syncopal episode. That is a medical word that means "we don't understand it."

The biggest concern was the fact that *the nurses were unable to obtain a pulse* (my italics) and they started cardiopulmonary resuscitation. The Emergency Room felt the patient needed to be observed to be sure that his cardiac status was stable."

Past, family and social history were unsatisfied. No complaints, no pain or lumps, denies shortage of breath and cough, denies chest pain, denies nausea and vomiting, etc.

Per Dr. Simon Dixon: stop taking Topcol (irregular heart); matter monitor next week (was not necessary); return to clinic in three months. Postmortem is my book, not an autopsy nor after death. That's it.

How, what, who, where? A BIG question…

What is a stroke?
Rich or poor, young or old. I will come after you. I can hit you so hard. I can paralyze an arm or leg. Or maybe, just maybe, I will kill you. I am a stroke. *(From American Stroke Association.)*

How do you have a stroke?
A stroke: it's a mark with a short line, to cancel by drawing a line through it; like a word in a sentence, according to the dictionary. Just the same thing, if you think about it. Medically, a sudden diminution or loss of consciousness, sensation and voluntary motion caused by rupture of obstruction of an artery of brain. It's called a brain attack or a stroke, which Hippocrates called the plesso, for "thunderstruck." The less common is hemorrhagic stroke, in which a blood vessel bursts causing bleeding into the brain. More commonly is ischemic stroke, which stalls from blood flowing blockage and causing a bleeding. Stroke is an equal threat to men and women, it occurs in all ages and races.

What is aphasia?
Consider it's the neurons that telegraph your brain through its communication – reading, writing and saying. It's the technical name

for interference with the comprehension and use of language. It results from brain injury or stroke. Sometimes aphasia develops from other condition in which the brain has been damaged. The first step in understanding is by recognizing that one problem, but a whole series of them. Every aphasic person is unique and must be treated as having a set of problems. Experts believe that aphasic people haven't actually lost their language, just their ability to recall and use it. Lots of patients can't recognize a single word or say a sound. After years, they can believe it and say them. Recovery doesn't mean learning like a child, but only recalling what they already know.

Is there a gene identified with stroke?

Researchers have identified a gene associated with increased risk for stroke. It has a stroke-susceptibility gene with has the greater risk of ischemic stroke, flowing the blood to brain and killing the cerebral tissue. The discovery will not lead to immediate treatments. However, the PDE4D gene, produces an enzyme that can be treated with drugs in the future.

How is it different from aphasia with apraxia?

Therapy repeats words and instruction on placement of oral structures. It teaches rhythm and rate, for example: using a metronome or finger-snapping to keep time, or prolonged duration of sentences. It produces the desired speech sound, contrary to aphasia which understand words, grammatical sentences and a connection with words and sentences. Aphasia finds the words to express a thought.

How do I have my job?

Maybe. The American Bar Association defines aphasia and presents case studies in which aphasia played a key role. Types of case is discussed in detail involve the competency of cases discussed in detail involve the competency of persons with aphasia to create and changes the ability of persons with aphasia. My job was significant from aphasia with absence of communication, especially with talking – conversing or interviewing – not really just writing. I was retired, at age of 49. Be real. Expect the employer for paying with your work. The Disability Rights Education and Defense Fund Hotline (800-466-4232) is funded by the Department of Justice. It will tell you if you can sue with your employer.

What's the difference between an occupation and occupational therapy?
As an editor, I had to find a thesaurus after years in my profession. I didn't know. It sounds like a good idea: occupational therapy helps you to live with your job. Not really. Moving, walking with a cane, or opening a door. They don't help you to perform your job or for your career. "Occupation" is a vocation, a business, an employment, a job. Occupational therapy is a term that is utilitarian, simply a function; anatomic, practical and necessary. It's a health-care profession that helps people with permanent, and temporary, disabilities from they can handle numerous physical problems; physical therapy or a physical instructor can be a slim chance with occupational therapy, but without any licenses or regulations. The emotional and mentally can benefit from occupational therapy. Physical therapists work to improve physical function and relieve pain using exercise, heat, cold and light therapy. Occupational therapists focus on the use of "meaningful activities" to restore function and independence. Coursework for a student includes liberal arts, anatomy and physiology, human development, health maintenance, psychology and others subjects.

What is speech and language therapy?
An only educator with a license or a degree can apply a speech and language therapy. The speech/language pathologist assists the stroke patient in relearning the communication skills necessary to rejoin his or her family, friends and colleagues.

What is Chapter 60: Equal Employment Opportunity?
A federal means equals contract the prohibition against discrimination in this part applies to the federal employment

activities: recruitment, advertising and job application procedures. Hiring, upgrading promotion, award of tenure, demotion, transfer, layoff, termination, right of return from layoff, and rehiring. Rates of pay or any other form of compensation and changes in compensation. Job assignments, job classifications, organizational structures, position descriptions, lines of progression, and seniority lists. Leaves of absences, sick leave, or any other leave, fringe benefits, selection and financial support for training.

How do I get the opportunities for disability?

One way is New Horizon, a United Way agency, approved by the Bureau of Worker's Disability Compensation. It's a private, not-for-profit organization founded in 1964. They can have employment services, but don't them to find you a job. You'll have to undertake it and coordinate, if you really want a job (work is a hard job!) Personnel who will assume all responsibility for training and supervision, and will coordinate transportation to and from the work site. Personnel who will be responsible for evaluating the consumers' performance and who are available to meet with the employer/employees as needed. They'll offer training and opportunities to develop life skills along with work skills. Coordinate with the Internet and emails; you still have links with associations. Don't forgive your friends, employees, etc. Volunteerism is a real opportunity; it's maybe a toe in the workplace.

What is a guardianship or conservators?

A guardian is a person who is appointed by a court to help to an individual make personal decisions when that person is unable to make such decisions. If a guardian is appointed for you, the guardian would make decisions for you that you now may make for yourself. For example, the guardian could decide such things as what medical care you receive and where you live. If appointed, the guardian will have the responsibility the secure service for you to restore you to the best possible state of mental and physical state well-being so that you can return to self-management at the earliest possible time. A person has been appointed by the court to more fully explain these matters to you. That person is called a guardian ad litem. He or she will contact you to those questions.

What is PABSS?

It is the Protection and Advocacy for Beneficiaries of Social Security, the "ticket to work" program. Over 70% of people with disabilities are unemployed. This program increases the incentives for people with disabilities to get and keep jobs. The ticket is like a voucher that lets you get employment services from agencies. It's voluntary – you won't go through the social security Continuing Disability Reviews while you are using your ticket. The trial work period allows you to test your ability to work for nine months in rolling a 60-month a period. You continue to be eligible for SSDI for 36 months after you successfully complete your trial work period. SSI checks continue until income exceeds limits. Medicare benefits up to 8 ½ years.

How do you get the drugs from money?

Marijuana doesn't help (just kidding). Canadian drug stores, available from the Internet, is a sticky but valuable tool. When medication is a necessary part of your total health care program, your health plan like Blue Cross, includes coverage for the following prescription drug services. You have coverage for federal and state-controlled drugs; pharmacists will automatically dispense the generic equivalent when appropriate if there is a generic equivalent to a brand name drug. Wholesale prices rose by 3.4% among the top 200 brand-name drugs while inflation was 1.2% in the first quarter of 2004.

What are nutraceuticals?

Don't help with "nutraceuticals" like garlic and seaweed. Experiment, if you like them, but as a supplement, not as medical from pharmaceuticals. An herb found in dozens of dietary supplements, sold as natural drugs advertised to lose weight and boost energy. There no long term, large scale study proving the herb's safety. Two ingredients in post-stroke life is aspirin (cheap!) and Plavix (see the book about it).

What exercises will help me?

Relax and warm your body. Remember to lie down, or modify the exercise as needed. Move through each joint's fullest range of motion without twisting or pulling yourself out of alignment. Exercising in front of a mirror may help you maintain good body posture. Each session should be performed two to four times a week. Weights are used to exercise even better: they can perform 40% a gain in overall strength, and 15% increased muscle mass to burning calories (25% increase of spontaneous exercise). They are used three times a week is recommended to minimize over training. Do 8 to 12 repetitions at first. Don't forget your arms, shoulders, hips, legs, thighs, backs and abdomen.

How do I nourish my marriage?

It's always better given with the pre-stroke marriage. Cherish it. Don't lose it. Many couples divorce after having a tough life. If your marriage is good, it will be happier with after a stroke. But if your marriage is bad… You can determine whether it's a benefit, or if it does not. Only one side can't have a marriage. I know that. Sorrow or sadness or pity won't help it. You'll see a happier life, maybe years after. It's not a preferred, more unplanned chance. But let her go. That's about all I can say. Don't expect anyone from questions and answers. You can ask them, or tell them what your position lies, but allow practice for your first choice. I'm not Dear Abby. I had a stroke. I have aphasia since then. I had a divorce, and I am not happy. But then, I will be happy later.

How do I plan or manipulate my life?

It's hard, with a pre-stroke and a complication with communications from aphasia. I didn't say I have no problems became having a stroke. Some of the stress triggers are traffic, work, money, marriage and illness. Stress is a natural part of daily living, and all of us experience it. Not everyone experiences that same level of stress or reacts to it in the same way. Recent medical evidence suggests a possible relationship between high levels of stress and increased risk of certain diseases, such as stroke. Take some precautions: take a therapy, a class, a meeting. If life is a problem before your stroke, it will be a bigger problem with your life after the stroke.

How can I get a scholarship or pay classes?

Look with adult enrichment at the community colleges or public education classes. Classes as only $99 per class for computers, yoga, gardening, or construction. Some seminars at the universities are free. Divorce workshops, jobs, anger, etc. all is out there. Ask a church, a singles group, a private-public partnership, or the county court. Time management, conflict resolution, balancing the home vs. career, budgeting and parents are seminars free. The Free Application for Federal Student Aid (FAFSA) is available from college or universities or at public libraries. It's harder to get any scholarships. Your disability means nothing. Unless you can learn from social security or the state occupational organization, they can offer classes: parenting, stress management, personal budgeting, rehabilitation services and math/reading brush-ups. You're almost better if you are getting your wallet for adult classes at community education.

What is transition?

Change happens in one of three ways: Imposed – not by choice; Gradually – allows time to adapt; Self-directed – by choice, actively make it happen. Self-directed change is your choice. Every change involves losses and gains. There are physical, intellectual or emotional changes.

What is cholesterol and what is wrong with it?

It's a member of family of molecules called lipids. They can't travel through blood in its original form because they don't mix with water. Most of cholesterol is in your body, made by the liver. Cholesterol means is very low-density lipoproteins (VLDL), low-density lipoproteins (LDL) and high-density lipoproteins (HDL). HDL returns cholesterol left in the blood vessels to the liver. VLDL carries fats to different parts of the body. LDL carries cholesterol to different parts of the body. If you eat too much fat, your liver makes extra VLDLs which eventually becomes LDLs. More cholesterol begins in the blood vessels. With 160 or more LDLs, you're good. In fact, you're having no heart disease and fewer than two risk factors other than high LDL cholesterol. If total cholesterol is greater than 200, or greater than 239 gives a borderline. Too much 240 g/ml is bad. Watch your weight. Stop smoking. Control your high blood pressure and diabetes. Drinking too much alcohol may raise the fat levels in your blood. Limit alcoholic beverages to no more than two each day. Exercise daily for your lifetime.

What are some dangerous risks?
Everybody knows weight, activity, smoking, high blood pressure, cholesterol and diabetes. Learn these new risks: infection, insulin resistance, C-reactive protein and homocysteine (it's almost cholesterol; it will clog your bloodstream). Infection is from a bacteria and viruses. Insulin resistance is not even with diabetes, but pre-diabetics. Whether insulin causes heart disease is unclear. C-reactive protein is associated with inflammation and a risk of stroke and heart attack

What do I earn for my disability?
Consider that in the thesaurus, disability means feebleness or impotent. Tell them it's not. Your disability benefits will continue as long as your condition has not medically improved and you cannot work. They will not necessarily continue indefinitely. More people with disabilities now recover from serious accidents and illnesses because of advances in medical science and rehabilitation techniques. Other people, through determination and effort, return to work in spite of serious conditions. As of January 2003, your benefits

will increase automatically if the cost of living has increased. If cost-of-living has increased by 2% during the year, your benefits will increase by 2%. The American with Disabilities Act will assess an individual's ability to work, and recommend adaptive equipment and workstation modifications. The statement of Employee Retirement Income Security Act (ERISA) rights is required by federal law and regulation.

Will I get or have my health benefits?

Ask your last employer. Mine has given me Blue Cross health benefits. Your employer may be better or worse. Ask them. If not, Medicare can be affected. The government's health insurance, it is for people age 65 or older, with disabilities who are under age 65 and people of any age who have permanent kidney failure. Medicare is financed by a portion of Federal Insurance Contributions Act (FICA) taxes, or payroll taxes, paid by workers and their employers. It also is financed in part by monthly premiums paid by beneficiaries. The Health Care Financing Administration is the agency in charge of the Medicare program. But the social security can help you enroll in the program and give you the general Medicare information.

How can I pay the mortgage for my house?

It's a big problem. Look at your life and what you live at your monthly money? Everybody has a budget. If you have a hospital fee, tell them you can do it in monthly bills. Give them $50, or $75 at the billing. Don't keep that $2,000 mortgage from your past home, but you can do it with a monthly rental or a cheaper condo/house. It's a harder life, I agree. But it only gets harder if you will grasp it sooner. Look at life with harder eyes, and a sharper pencil. Your life is hard, harder when you are making money and a job (*your* job). Car insurance, utilities, groceries, etc. can be skinnier with a slimmer budget. Consider your budget, and ask yourself: can I pay with two dollars from a dollar? Can you turn into a penny pincher? I can do it and you can do it, too.

How do I talk to my sons and daughters?

As parents, we have a common bond among our children. To help children grow into responsible adults. To raise a child who is loved and able to give love. Expect them to give a choice, if they're 7 or 8 or 9. If they're something bad, it was for some attention, power, revenge, or display of inadequacy. Don't always set a model, if they're 15 or 16 ages plus. Children get messages from you, a parent. They'll be children, all ages and all stages. They won't listen. But, in case, they will listen and pay attention, if it's they still are unnoticed or carelessness. Keep it simple. Send them a greeting card, a card for *un*-birthdays. Give him/her a verse from a poem or a rock song if they are at college. Maybe a joke, a short story. Email them a single, well-thought sentence or a paragraph. It doesn't have a long discussion. It really should not be an insurance policy or a treatise written by a lawyer. They should write: love, Dad (or Mom). That tells about it.

*And now, another word (at least **one!**)...*

Developing the courage to be imperfect. It's true. Children will have happy, confident, cooperative and responsible, according to the *Parents Handbook*. You can do it, wrongly. A parent is infallible, but they can be trustworthy. Don't give it time. Don't ever give it up.

How do I ask her (him) for a date?

Make a letter. Or even better, use email. You get an idea, and write it on ink. The correct words (spelling and thesaurus with computer or books) will be there, on paper or electronic. Think it about a second or third reading. Don't SEND the email unless it is sure exactly what you try to send. You can edit it, delete it, anything you want. With the phone or with personal one-to-one conversations, I can do it with a word, or two words, or three. Nod your head. Smile. Say uuuummmm-hmmmm. Don't let it gone. Don't be a mute or a mimic. Use a gesture. Don't try to say it, if it's going to 10 or 15 words in a sentence. You'll be crazy, stammering or muttering, and saying the wrong words. I know. Don't write too much. Just your name, maybe your age and address, and tell them what you would like to have a dinner, or a social date like a baseball game or a movie. "Ed, Thank you so much for asking me to dinner… I'm glad to see you are doing so well after having a stroke. I hope to remain friends with you. Deborah." It's exactly from a personal card. Don't tell them everything about your stroke, the doctors and the hospitalization. It's boring. And they don't care!

How can I still have sex? How often?
As many as you can. Continue pre-stroke hobbies and activities as much as possible. Said one survivor, her husband said he could not have a person with disability with sex. She wanted it. She divorced him. I'm looking for a wife, a girlfriend, etc. A trade magazine tells us: "Go to the mall or grocery store with your survivor so you both can enjoy some physical activity." Well, not have sex at the grocery store. Well, maybe even at the grocery store… in the produce section, not the frozen foods.

What is the future for me?
There is an answer. A new generation of neuropharmacology presents improved memory or cognitive performance "in impaired individuals" (not my wording) are under intensive testing. The vision would deliver drugs that would stimulate the train to replace its own cells. There is a stem cell operation that can repair or produce new neurons. Promising without drugs or operations begins with transcranial magnetic stimulation (TMS), which can repair brain tissue. A magnetic field can safely penetrate and activate the brain's inner regions and generate stimulation neurons. They are noninvasive (safely) for brains and potential offers many applications.

What do I communicate with aphasia?
Listen comprehension. I will be "overloaded" with television or fast talkers. It may appear when she/he doesn't understand. Read comprehension. It may not understand letters, words, sentences and/ or directions. Readers may not remember what has just been read. Their desire must be lost or missed. Verbal expression. Words may

sound slurred or not completely express ideas. Written expression. He/she may be have problems of spelling or write the wrong words. Sentences will have shorter – "but", "and", "with" conjunctions are not common. Five and seventy five cents is $5.75. Ninety equals 90. Maybe it does not compute with a patient with aphasia.

How do I daily live with aphasia?

Take classes. Talk to therapists, psychologists, social security or job counselors. Talk or email instructors, or read everything you want to learn. If you can't read, writers can be books on tape or VHS or computer diskettes/CD-ROMs. Ask them what you have questions. Patients are among the best people. Go to meetings. Your friends, family is (sometimes!) knowledgeable. Don't ASK them: *ask* them what you should do; don't expect them to be a guru or a coach. If you ask them, they'll answer – a big, bad, thoughtfully reason. Because there will be a monitor, sometimes a protégé. Ask them what they say, and forget it. You aren't a child. You're an adult. Believe your life. You have a voice. Use it. You have a say-so or have an opinion. As always, take your own voice: give it a barkin' dog!

How can I tell them with aphasia?

Emails, letters and talking... with dictionaries and thesaurus. Consider learning a laptop or desktop computer, if you don't already have one. A Franklin Electronic Merriam-Webster's Collegiate Dictionary costs $99. It costs more than a printed book, but less than a computer. The speaking version also supports line of electronic books and pronounces words and short sentences. It's handy and portable. It includes all 200,000 words from the print edition. It's not for only aphasia patients. It's for students and writers and everyone who needs a dictionary – *everyone.* If you're not sure how to pronounce "phat" just press the button with the picture of a speaker on it. A computer will speak the word as clearly as your speech-language therapist. It's about 3 pounds and comprised 1,165 pages. Of course, it will pronounce the words "bitch" and "bastard," but not pronounce the word "fuck." You're on your own!

What is the future for strokes or aphasia?
For now, there are drugs that may be helpful. Epidermal growth factors (EGF) and fibroblast growth factors (FGF) are being used to enhance this neuron's repairing process. They are large molecules, unfortunately, crossing with the blood-brain barrier. Aricept, manufacturers by Eisai Inc. and Pfizer Inc., helps human genes that predisposed to Alzheimer's abnormalities in neurogenesis. The left temporal lobe and thalamus are specialized for language and speech memories, while the right temporal lobe and thalamus for seeing and viewing memories. Prozac, an anti-depression drug, manipulates neurogenesis in experimental animals. Most of them take up to one month for mood – the same time required for neurogenesis. But long term administration of antidepressants appears to spur neurogenesis. Amphetamines (like caffeine) may help also. Normal, healthy adults can handle amphetamines with improved alertness. Amphetamines like modafinil or caffeine (or coffee), and depression-preventive symptoms like Provac or Valium, or even dopamine (L-dopa) can survive and alert the neurons.

What is a Cosmopolitan?
Add an ounce of orange vodka, ½ ounce of Courvasier and a splash of cranberry juice (just in case).

Appendix

Shortly, after the stroke, I was giving a picture and I would say a word. It's hard, if you just had a stroke. It's awful, frightful, unbearing, demeaning and degraded. But it has, as it goes, to walk rather than one runs. A picture of a fork. What do you eat with it? Or the picture of a pencil or a clock. An aphasic might say "lamp" when he's got a vision with a telephone. The therapist tells "touch my ear," and the aphasic patient might think that means an ear, but it doesn't tell the same thing. He touches his nose. The patient can carefully watch for the therapist, seeing their lips and gesturing their hands.

Synonyms

The synonyms are relevant to therapy. There are my words that make them sense to my thinking.

lazy – indifference, lax opposite of work

haunted – a spooky ghost; frightened, scary

damp – moist, wet; mold inhibits; opposite of desert, arid

pretend – act to

graceful – thankful

prevent – to prohibit

scrub – to clean using a brush or a sponge

nervous – making it upset, jittery

miracle – wish

bitter – sour or distaste

tickle – puts him a giggle

apologize – sorry, a showing of remorse

surprise – shock, welcome

fancy – rich, showing style; not poor

germs – microbes that are unhealthy

deny – not right, incorrect

dizzy – faint, unconscious

fiction – not possible; play-being; not truth

impossible – not able, not possible

secret – sssssssh! confidential, not aware of plans

Antonyms
Another favorite! Some people (aphasics and others) can read synonyms, but can't find antonyms, like the opposite or contrasts.
Hate – love
Cold – hot
Peace – war
Caution –unwary
Brave – timid, uncourageous
Soft – hard
Hardcover book – softcover book
Accelerate – brake, decelerate
Freeze – boil, heat, melt
Thank you – critical, unappreciative
Republican – Democrat
Conservative – liberal

Fill in the appropriate category member
Holiday, vegetables, units of measure, names
C – Christmas, corn, centimeter, Carol
G – George Washington President, gourd, gigameter, George
T – Thanksgiving, tomatoes, tenths, Tony
S – St. Pat's Day, squash, semi-, Stanley
Cities, colors, fruits, animals
B – Boston, brown, blueberry, bull
P – Philadelphia, pink, plum, peacock
F – Fort Worth, fuscia, fig, fly
G – Green Bay, green, grapes, grasshopper

Scrambled sentences:
The candlesticks   are made of pewter.
I would like to   have a glass of wine.
My pants aretoo long.
Ham and eggs   are good for breakfast.
Was have lived in Troy   for seven years.
I want to   see him elected chairman.

The Bicentennial was   in 1976.
World War II ended in 1945.
Columbus discovered America   in 1492.
She needs to frost   the chocolate cake.
He needs to wash   the windows.
He needs to read   the instructions.

Word recall

Can the patient identify a brand name, as someone can call a single or double words like the word "I'd like a cup of Maxwell House" instead of coffee, and "I'd like a Pepsi, please?" Does anyone really say, "I'd like a soft drink, maybe a brown sugar cola?" Can a brand name is differed with a generic word, like with "Kleenex" comes up instead of "facial tissue"? Maybe they'll "drive the car to Farmer Jack's" rather than "drive the car to the supermarket." They can be the first words that are spoken!

    toothpaste – Crest, Colgate, Pepsodent

    ice cream – Breyer's, Good Humor, Edy's

    shoes – Florsheim, Nike, Adidas, Ascis, Timberland

    beer – Labatt's, Molson, Rolling Rock, Budweiser, Samuel Adams (I could take an hour!)

    coffee – Maxwell House, Folgers, Starbucks

    soft drink – Coke, Pepsi, Mountain Dew, Sprite

    cereal – Kellogg, General Mills, Cheerios, Froot Loops (brand names or companies)

    raincoat – London Fog (just the one?)

Write the name of the place where you would find each of the items listed: Mt. Fuji, Japan; Cape Cod, Mass. It was easy, for me. I had visited almost state, because of my travels. Cities in Ohio, Illinois, Florida, New York. There was a clear and neat scene in my mind. And I was near the therapy and almost was "plateauing". It sounded the first month of therapy: Monday, Tuesday, Wednesday; January, February, March. I had a tough job at speaking and pronouncing August – my own birthday! Even also the alphabet, and numbers – 0, 1, 2, 3, 4. Therapy begins at the starting. First grade.

Calendar and date for today, and their birth date. Aphasics must take them on first, second and third. We can take them for granted. For locations are fun: The Everglades, Florida. Niagara Falls, Ontario, Canada. Taj Mahal, India. Buckingham Palace, England.

Word power

karaoke – a) canoe b) martial arts c) singing d) nightclub

cocooning – a) *staying at home* b) oversleeping c) knitting d) making silk

tree hugger – a) South American frog b) *environmentalist* c) many-winged insect d) arborist's tool

pathography – a) study of tropical diseases b) sports medicine c) *biography* (on the negative elements of a subject, the study of the effects of illness on a historical person's life) d) x-rays

fashionista – who is a) *clothing-savvy* b) a designer c) a right-winger d) intriguing

agita – a) *anxiety or agitation* b) fright c) restlessness d) harmony

bork – a) to hit b) jump over c) *attack* d) fasten (To attack someone, especially in the media. From Judge Robert Bork, whose nomination to the Supreme Court was blocked by negative information – can I make up such a word?)

wannabe – a) one who takes identities b) has aspirations c) studies kangaroos d) angry

Memory recall

Four unrelated words, for example:

Sometimes bridge move scary

Blue happy tall enjoy

Next further still pond

Four words, including a verb, a noun, a pronoun – it doesn't matter but not just four concrete nouns. It's harder when you gather them in four different words! Make them a single syllable and two syllables or three. Make them tougher!

Then try them to gather four numbers or four digits:

5, 8, 4, 1

9, 7, 8, 4

Make them harder if they're not in sequence: 1, 4, 5, 8.

Next, try two digits and one digit numbers: 16, 4, 39, 31. Then try five numbers. It's hard even when you've not had a stroke and/or aphasia! Seven digits from an answering machine: the telephone number is 983-3907. It's easier or more complicated when the area code is also a number. Maybe you can understand if it's an area code; my phone numbers usually are three area codes: 313, 586, and 248. Makes it harder when the voice is quicker or slurred, isn't it? If you have a phone answering machine, get the first time you get the phone numbers. Remember if you don't, rerun again.

Sentence construction

A dog walked by. It was a black dog.

A black dog walked by.

It was a cloudy afternoon. It was cool.

It was a cloudy, cool afternoon.

It was a cloudy, cool afternoon with raining during the evening.

That's really a way of making single sentences. Now, I was ready at the time, trying to short sentences, without "and" and "but." I can do it. I shortened my writing, with the help with my therapist. I can do it, shortening my writing. Do you write a lead paragraph with the idea of 25 or 30 words? You shouldn't! A reader won't read the too-long. Are your media similar to newspapers, or Scientific American? Fifth grade or master of science? There can be a difference.

Frequently misspelled words

Accommodate

Specialty

Hemorrhage

Tariff

Spaghetti

Seizure

Aneurysm

Aphasia

Buffet

Zucchini
Simile
Pickles
Annul
Annually

Get your own list: 100 or 200 or 1,000 words. It's harder without having a case of aphasia!

Finish each sentence

Run the _____ (track).
Close the _____ (door).
Look at the _____ (cat running the dog).
Jump over the _____ (fence).
What _____ (time) is it?
Is it the time to _____ (go).
Wash the _____ (car with a bucket and a sponge).
Open your _____ (window).
Turn off the _____ (lights).

Sentence construction

I like _____ because _____.

I don't the end like this one. Because it can be everything – I like ice cream because it's good.

I don't like _____ because _____. I don't like orange Jell-O because it tastes evil and tastes chemical.

Explain what each word means by describing it or telling how it's used (similar to a synonym, it the writer has a vocabulary). The patient can five or six words without making a 12 or 14 or 16 in a sentence – and making him or she wandering like in a swamp!

Belt – You wear a belt to hold up your pants.

Pen – You write with a pen. A pen has blue ink.

Hot dog – He ate for lunch. He ate a hot dog.

Punctuation

Punctuation was a favorite for me. I was born with it. I read the comics and cereal box. A word with its misspelling, question mark for sentences, double negatives, – it makes me, as an editor, as mad (like insanity or craziness)!

where do you live – Where do you live?

it seemed as though the time would never pass – It seemed as though the time would never pass.

Word power

Avoid using a $5 word when a 50 cents word will do. But during this, we offer that can embellish your conversation or correspondence (like your time with a non-friend or non-family like a business acquaintance):

brouhaha – hubbub, uproar; A brouhaha in a crowd.

feckless – ineffective; incompetent; having no sense of responsibility ingratiate – to seek favor by getting into someone's good graces; as You'd be wise to ingratiate yourself with the new boss.

syncline – in structural geology a rock fold in which the stratum dips toward the central axis, like a trough.

panache – (have you ever given this one?) flamboyance; grand manner also a plume of feathers or tassels on a helmet.

preen – primp; dress smartly; birds of cleaning and preening to the feathers with the beak.

quotidian – everyday; recurring daily as stockholders and eager for their quotidian market reports.

serendipity – luck in finding something accidentally, as the serendipity of getting the first job you apply for.

donnybrook – a rowdy brawl; as in a fight at a saloon or in a crowd.

chortle – to chuckle gleefully; to sing or chant exultantly.

grock – to understand, to know (a word by science fiction author Robert Heinlein)

fensity – "almost" Christmas holiday (as seen in Jerry Seinfeld sitcom)

(Want to pick your own words? Allow me; it's easy!)

Scrambled sentence

Unscramble the words and put them in the correct order to form a sentence. My hardest one. If I can get this one, I feel I'm almost perfect, almost 100%. After you get the results, or you don't get the results either, make it to try the next time. A day or so may be the sentence correct.

sun today the is shining – Today, the sun is shining.

find can't my sweater I – I can't find my sweater.

end street a this is dead – This end is a dead street.

time leave what we should – What time should we leave?

I am the world's smallest giant. I am the world's largest giant.

I turned the radio on so that I could watch the movie. I turned the t.v. on so that I could watch the movie.

The bases were loaded so they attempted a field goal. The bases were loaded so they attempted a squeeze bunt.

I shut the book and started reading. I opened the book and started reading.

The ink in my pencil ran out. The ink in my pen ran out.

Morphemic usage part I

I went (to) the store.

I have five fingers (on) each hand.

She set the table (with) diner.

I opened the bottle (with) a can opener.

We went out to dinner (and) there was nothing (to) eat in the house.

He cut the meat (with) a knife.

She weighed the vegetables (on) the scale.

I bought candy (at) the store.

Morphemic usage part II

She _____ (can, *is*, are, has) twelve years old.

I _____ (has begun, begun, *began*, did begun) to get ready to leave.

Both you and I _____ (*were,* was, is, has) planning to go to the movies.

I'm tired of _____ (*sitting,* setting, setting, has sat) in this chair.

Please _____ (lay, lie, lain, lied) down and take a nap.

If you _____ (listen, are listening, has listened, was listening) to me, you wouldn't have gotten lost.

The boys _____ (swum, had swimmed, *swam,* had swam) out to the dock.

If you want me to, I _____ (sent, send, have sent, *will send*) you a replacement.

I'm tired of sitting/setting/satting/has sat in this chair *(sitting).*

Both you and I were/was/is/has planning to go to the movies *(were).*

Spatial relations

Materials: Cut from pictures from newspapers or magazines

Task instructions: Arrange stimulus materials in two rows of five. Place the pictures in the following order. First row (for example): bell, radio, umbrella, kite, saw. Second row: tent, pipe, refrigerator, automobile, flashlight.

Clinician instruments: "I'm going to have you do some things with certain objects. Listen carefully and do just what I tell you to do."

Suggested criteria: 90% accuracy without the need of repetition of the task instructions or significant delays in responding.

Put the bell to the left of the radio.

Put the umbrella to the right of the kite.

Put the saw between the tent and pipe.

Put the automobile to the left of the refrigerator.

And so on…

Temporal relations

Materials: Cut from pictures from newspapers or magazines.

Task instructions: Arrange the stimulus items in two rows of five.

Clinician instructions: "I'm going to have you do some things with each of these. Listen carefully and do just what I tell you to do."

Suggested criteria: 90% accuracy without the need of repetition of the task instructions or significant delays in responding.

After I nod my head, pick up the spoon.

Touch the cup after I raise my hand.

Before I look at the ceiling, pick up the phone

After I point to you, turn over the watch.

And so on…

Make up a sentence using each word

Cup – Eight ounces in a cup.

Read – Read and write this story.

Hungry – When it is time for dinner, I am hungry.

Get – Get along, little doggies!

Who – Who is there?

Medicine – This medicine will make me well.

Dime – A dime is 10 cents, and less than a dollar.

Under – The car was underneath the bridge in a tunnel.

Stupid – This sentence is stupid!

Glossary

Aggrenox – trademark; reduces the stroke as aspirin and antiplatelet such as Plavix or Ticlid.

Aneurysm – an abnormal thinning and protrusion of a blood vessel wall caused when the lining becomes weakened and expands in size. It poses a risk of rupturing and bleeding.

Anomia – in the vernacular of clinical aphasia refers both to a specific clinical sign and a clinical syndrome

Anticoagulants – medications that prevent blood clotting.

Aphasia – loss or impairment of the power to use or comprehend words usually resulting from brain damage. Group of disorders of language arising from disease or damage to the brain; a person has problems formulating or comprehending speech and difficulty in reading and writing.

Apraxia – term for a disorder of articulation in which there is obvious difficulty initiating utterances, articulatory inconsistency, and effortful grouping.

Aspirin – a white crystalline derivative of acetysalicyclic acid used for relief of pain and fever; can cause allergic reaction but also a drug for strokes and heart disease.

Botox – (botulinum toxic type A) trademark by Allergen Inc. approved by U.S. Food and Drug Administration to smooth certain wrinkles on the face, may help some stroke survivors regain use of clenched and rigid hands.

Brain attack – describes the action and effect of a stroke on the brain.

Brain imaging – techniques to help to define brain function or determine the severity of brain damage.

Brain stem – stalk-like portion of the brain in vertebrates that includes everything except the cerebellum and the cerebral hemispheres. It provides a channel for all signals passing between the spinal cord and the higher parts of the brain.

Broca's aphasia – the nonfluent speech of individuals with aphasia to be contracted with the fluent speech of Wernicke's aphasia.

Cardiovascular – relating to the heart and blood vessels.

Cerebellum – second largest division of the brain. Controls coordination of voluntary movements including walking, talking, and most play activities require coordination.

Computed tomography – CT, a computerized scanning technique that uses X-ray pictures to create cross-sectional images of the brain or other organs from many different angles. Also, computerized axial tomography (CAT), used widely in the 1970s.

Conduction aphasia – hypothesized with Wernicke the existence of a distinct type of aphasia based on his neuroanatomic model of language localization of the brain.

Coumadin – Commonly used anticoagulant, used called warfarin.

Dopamine – one of the most important neutrotransmitters, it has a healthy level which makes you feel good. But too much or too little can it cause problems. They can involve schizophrenia, Parkinson's disease, depression etc.

Embolism – sudden blocking of a vessel by an embolus; one cause of ischemic stroke.

Electroencephalography (EEG) – one of the oldest examining technologies from 1875, it can detect your brain's electrical signals; its sensors record this information.

Electroconvulsive therapy (ECT) – a procedure in which electrodes are attached to the scalp, the best of them but remain somewhat problematic for various reasons. They are nonfocal; can lead to memory side effects, and require repeated general anesthesia.

Hemiparesis – Weakness on one side of the body.

Hemorrhagic – a stroke that occurs when a blood vessel ruptures in or near the brain.

High density lipoprotein (HDL) – the cholesterol called the "good" because it helps your body get of bad cholesterol.

Hippocampus – deep in the brain near the temporal lobe part of the lateral ventricles. They are important from a speech-language and memory with words.

Infarction – area of tissue in an organ that has died.

Ischemic – a stroke that occurs when part of the brain is suddenly deprived of blood.

Lipitor – drug trademark by Pfizer Inc. to reduce cholesterol for heart disease.

Lipoprotein – fat, protein. Fat is hooked up to protein in the blood and is carried in the blood as lipoprotein.

Low density lipoprotein (LDL) – the protein that carries the bad cholesterol in the blood.

Magnetic resonance imaging (MRI) – a computerized scan technique that uses magnetic fields to create images of internal organs. By measuring blood flow, a type of MRI called fMRI (functional MRI) can show how the brain works during specific activities.

Magnetic seizure therapy (MST) – a supercharged version of TMS, they can produce beneficial seizures in depressed patients.

Neurologist – a physician experienced in the diagnosis and treatment of the nervous system.

Neurons – basic structural unit of the nervous system that enables rapid transmission of impulses between different parts of the body. Electrical messages travel 220 miles or 323 feet per second! They are long, spidery cells with arms like tentacles.

Nonvalvular atrial fibrillation (NVAF) plaque – deposits of fatty material in the arteries.

Plavix (trademark) – helps blood platelets from sticking together and forming clots, helping raise your protection against future heart attack of stroke. Manufactured by Bristol-Meyers Squibb Co.

Platelets – smallest of three types of cells in the blood.

Positron emission tomography (PET) – provided of color photos of brain activity, such as speaking, listening or the patient is learning as looking at pictures. To do a PET scan, scientists inject safe but detectable amounts of radioactive chemicals into a person's bloodstream.

Pravachol (trademark) – a prescribed drug to see if you haven't reduced cholesterol due to diet and exercise. Pravachol (pravastatin sodium) made by Bristol-Myers Squibb Co.

Stent – a drug-coated to stop the growth of unwanted tissue from plugging up the blood vessel as said to be reliable as a heart bypass operation

Stress – constraining force or influence. A physical, chemical or emotional factor that causes a bodily or mental tension and may be a factor in disease causation.

Stroke – a sudden loss in function of a part of the brain caused by interference with its blood supply.

Thrombus – a blood clot that forms inside a blood vessel.

Transient doppler (TCD) ultrasound – an effective way to safely study blood flow in the arteries.

Transient ischemic attack (TIA) – a mini-stroke whose symptoms resemble ischemic stroke but disappear within 24 hours; often an imminent or warning signs of stroke.

Transcranical magnetic stimulation (TMA) – a noninvasive technique using head-mounted wire coils that send strong but very brief magnetic pulses directly into specific brain regions, inducing tiny electric currents in a person's neural circuitry.

Ultrasound – Sonographers look for plaque in the main arteries leading to the brain. Excessive fatty plaque builds in the carotid arteries increasing your stroke.

Warfarin (Coumadin) – decrease the tendency in heart attacks and strokes of blood making a clot.

Zocor (trademark) – drug to dramatically lower LDL cholesterol and increasing the HDL (good cholesterol.) Made by Merck Inc.

Zoloft (trademark) – an anti-stress tablet contains sertaline hydrochloride to 50mg, made by Pfizer U.S. Pharmaceuticals.

Books, magazines, videocassettes and manuals

(By no means, but these are the only ones I have researched on my book)

American Heart Association, *Family Guide to Stroke Treatment, Recovery, and Prevention* by Louis R. Caplan, MD, Random House Inc., New York, 1994.

Aphasia and Related Neurogenic Language Disorders by Leonard L. LaPointe, Arizona State University, Thieme Medical Publishers, New York.

Assessment and Management of Emotional and Psychosocial Reactions to Brain Damage and Aphasia by Peter Wahrborg, Singular Publishing Corp.

Brain Attack by Paulina Perez and Marsha Rehns, Cutting Edge Press, a division of Perez Enterprises Inc.

Communication: Aphasia, a pamphlet by the Home Care Companion, 888-846-7008 (VC).

Coping with Aphasia by Jon G. Lyon, Singular Publishing Corp.

DNA, The Secret of Life by James D. Watson, Random House Inc.

Fact Sheet by National Aphasia Association, a four-page summary. National Aphasia Association, 351 Butternut Ct., Millersville, MD 21108.

'I Need Help': A Stroke Patient's Plea by Helen Underwood, Blue Dolphin Publishing.

Pathways; Moving Beyond Stroke and Aphasia by Susan Adair Ewing and Beth Pfalgraf, Wayne State University Press; 1990.

Portrait of Aphasia by David Knox, Wayne State University Press; 1971 third printing in 1985.

Recovering at Home After a Stroke: A Practical Guide for You & Your Family by Florence Weiner, Berkley Publishing Group, New York, 1994.

Striking Back At Stroke by Cleo Hutton and Louis R. Caplan, MD, The Dana Press, Washington DC, 2003.

The Serper Method of Brain Recovery, Regrowth and Vitality by Lynn Serper from Brain Enhancement Services Inc., 1501Beacon Street, Suite 1606, Brookline, MA 02446.

Stroke, by Lawrence M. Brass, MD.

Stroke Connection magazine by American Stroke Association

Stroke Smart magazine by the National Stroke Association

Stroke: at Time of Diagnosis; TimeLife Medical (VC); and a handy pamphlet

The Male Stress Survival Guide by Georgia Witkin, PhD, Newmarket Press, New York.

Working With Apraxic Clients; A Practical Guide to Therapy for Apraxia, by Susan Huskin, Communication Skill Builders.

The Writers Handbook; an article "Writers: See How They're Run" by Joyce Carol Oates

Associations and Organizations

American Heart Association (AHA)
7272 Greenville Ave.
Dallas, TX 75231-4596
800-553-6321
www.americanheart.org

American Academy of Neurology
1080 Montreal Avenue
St. Paul, MN 55116
651-695-1940
www.aan.com

American Speech-Language-Hearing Association
10801 Rockville Pike
Rockville, MD 20852
301-897-5700; 800-638-8255
www.asha.org

Brain Attack Coalition
(A group of several stroke associations including professions, volunteers and government agencies.)
www.stroke-site.org

National Institute of Neurological Diseases and Stroke
P.O. Box 5801
Bethesda, MD 20824
800-352-9424
www.ninds.nih.gov/health

National Stroke Association
8480 East Orchard Rd. Suite 1000
Englewood, CO 80111-5015
800-787-6537
www.stroke.org

National Aphasia Association
156 Fifth Avenue, Suite 707
New York, NY 10010
212-255-4329 or 800-922-4622
www.aphasia.org

National Rehabilitation Information Center
8455 Colesville Rd. Suite #935
Silver Spring, MD 20910-3319
800-346-2742

Manufactured By: RR Donnelley
Momence, IL USA
October, 2010